An Occupational Perspective on Leadership

Theoretical and Practical Dimensions

An Occupational Perspective on Leadership

Theoretical and Practical Dimensions

Sandra Barker Dunbar, DPA, OTR/L, FAOTA
Professor, Occupational Therapy Department
Nova Southeastern University
Fort Lauderdale, FL

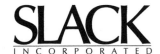

SLACK
INCORPORATED

www.slackbooks.com

ISBN: 978-1-55642-873-9

The Instructor's Manual is also available from SLACK Incorporated. Don't miss this important companion to *An Occupational Perspective on Leadership: Theoretical and Practical Dimensions*. To obtain the Instructor's Manual, please visit http://www.efacultylounge.com.

Published by: SLACK Incorporated
                 6900 Grove Road
                 Thorofare, NJ 08086 USA
                 Telephone: 856-848-1000
                 Fax: 856-848-6091
                 www.slackbooks.com

Contact SLACK Incorporated for more information about other books in this field or about the availability of our books from distributors outside the United States.

Library of Congress Cataloging-in-Publication Data

An occupational perspective on leadership : theoretical and practical dimensions / [edited by] Sandra Barker Dunbar.
    p. ; cm.
  Includes bibliographical references and index.
  ISBN 978-1-55642-873-9 (alk. paper)
  1. Occupational therapy--Administration. 2. Leadership. I. Dunbar, Sandra Barker
  [DNLM: 1. Occupational Therapy--organization & administration. 2. Leadership. 3. Professional Role. WB 555 O14029 2009]
  RM735.4.O225 2009
  615.8'515--dc22
                            2009012128

Printed in the United States of America.

Last digit is print number: 10   9   8   7   6   5   4   3   2   1

Dedication

This book is dedicated to Marty Breyer, OTR/L and Debbie Holmes Enix, MPH, OTR/L, my mentors who exemplified stellar leadership.

Contents

Acknowledgments

The authors acknowledge the respective leaders in our lives who have challenged our thinking, supported our personal and professional growth, and paved the way for innovative practice.

About the Editor

Sandra (Sandee) Barker Dunbar completed her undergraduate degree at Loma Linda University in Loma Linda, CA, her master of arts in occupational therapy from New York University in New York City, and her doctor of public administration degree from Nova Southeastern University in Fort Lauderdale, FL. The latter degree exposed her to organizational behavior, leadership, management, and strategic planning content, all of which have influenced her work in occupational therapy.

She currently teaches leadership content on both the masters and doctoral levels of education at Nova Southeastern University as part of her occupational role as professor. She has also held several management and leadership positions in clinical and academic settings throughout her years in the occupational therapy profession. Sandee enjoys mentoring activities, including this project with Nova Southeastern University doctoral students who participated in her Leadership course.

Contributing Authors

Tara Beitzel, MA, OTR/L (Chapter 3)
Assistant Professor, Occupational Therapy Program
The University of Findlay
Findlay, OH

Marge E. Boyd, MPH, OTR/L (Chapter 4)
Faculty Coordinator, Academics & Fieldwork
Research Faculty
Occupational Therapy Program
Dominican College
Orangeburg, NY

Jan G. Garbarini, MA, OTR/L (Chapter 2)
Assistant Professor
Research Coordinator
Occupational Therapy Program
Dominican College
Orangeburg, NY

Tami Lawrence, MS, OTR/L (Chapter 4)
Owner, Hilton Head Pediatric Therapy Center
Hilton Head Island, SC

Teresa Plummer, MSOT, OTR, ATP (Chapter 5)
Instructor, School of Occupational Therapy
Belmont University
Nashville, TN

Laura Schmelzer, MOT, OTR/L (Chapter 3)
Assistant Professor, Occupational Therapy Program
The University of Findlay
Findlay, OH

Lesly S. Wilson, PhD, OTR/L (Chapter 6)
Research Assistant Professor
University of South Carolina
Center for Disability Resources
Team for Early Childhood Solutions (TECS)
Columbia, SC

Foreword

People live and work in groups, and this has been key to our development and survival as a species since the dawning of time. We are social animals, and we must cooperate in order to assure our safety and mutual advantage.[1] But we have also learned that by working together, we can accomplish much more than as individuals. We can achieve great dreams, even to the point now that we are able to explore the universe beyond our planet. Contemplation of this remarkable progress reveals how truly extraordinary and powerful cooperation can be.

The idea of groups of people working together for shared benefit and common purpose is fundamental to the idea of organization, or assigning structure and purpose to groups. McNamara defined an organization as "a group of people intentionally organized to accomplish an overall common goal or set of goals."[2] Organizations may be simple and consist of few people, or they can be complex with thousands of people operating at a global level. Regardless of their size or complexity, however, they all have one thing in common: to work most effectively, they need leadership.

In primitive times, leaders evolved informally based on family membership, strength, age, or popularity. While some leaders were benevolent and wise, others were ruthless and ignorant. Power was based on position, and the only leadership training was that attained vicariously or learned on the job. Great power was assumed to equate to great leadership. Fast forward to the 21st century. We now know that leading people effectively requires more than family heritage or armies of ten thousand warriors. We understand that effective leadership is both an art and a science. We know that specific skills can be learned and applied to influence groups toward desired ends, and we understand that leadership is required in every organization.

As professionals, occupational therapists are accustomed to working in organizations, as members of teams, and in communities, each of which are groups of people with a shared interest in particular outcomes or sets of goals. Learning about effective leadership is a highly appropriate topic for the profession. This is one of the reasons why I have been interested throughout my professional career in studying leadership, attempting to apply its principles, and in advocating for leadership development within the profession.[3] In my present role, it brings me great satisfaction that the American Occupational Therapy Foundation recognizes the vital importance of leadership development to the future of the profession, and actively supports programs that address this essential need.

The education of occupational therapists provides a strong foundation upon which to build in developing effective leaders. Knowledge of people, tasks, groups, and systems provides a useful beginning, but truly effective leadership requires a keen knowledge of principles, abundant practice, communication skills, character, and the right values. To be a good leader, one must also know how to be a good follower, a dedicated and tenacious student, and a servant who is dedicated to causes beyond the self.

I am pleased that Sandee Dunbar has assembled such a talented group of authors to write this book. It is comprehensive, it is relevant, and it is contemporary. It addresses the important theories, principles, and values of leadership in a readable, competent, and practical manner. Its collective messages contribute in significant ways to the literature of occupational therapy. More importantly, if it contributes to the development of even one more effective leader, it has met its purpose, thereby demonstrating an important message this book emphasizes: leadership helps groups attain collective goals.

Charles H. Christiansen, EdD, OTR, OT(C), FAOTA
Executive Director
The American Occupational Therapy Foundation
Bethesda, Maryland

References

1. Dawkins R. *The Selfish Gene*. 2nd ed. Oxford, UK: Oxford University Press; 1989.
2. McNamara C. Free Management Library. 2006. Available at http://www.managementhelp.org. Accessed August 9, 2006.
3. Christiansen C. Leadership skills. In: Duncan EAS, ed. *Skills for Practice in Occupational Therapy*. London, UK: Churchill Livingson; 2008.

Introduction

Theory provides the foundation for a profession's frames of reference and models. Occupational therapy is no exception to this rule. The profession has long recognized the value of systematically identifying these guideposts that enable us to be called true professionals. The distinction between professions can relate to the theoretical underpinnings that clearly delineate areas of concern. Developmental, behavioral, and psychosocial theories are just a few of the types of basic theoretical areas that the occupational therapy profession has drawn from. Clearly, these contributions have enhanced our guides to practice in working with children and adults. They have also enabled us to develop and maintain professional status.

With an appreciation for how theory has enhanced our professionalism as occupational therapists, it is an easy transition to accept that the application of leadership theories can also enhance our practice. The application of leadership theories can improve one's ability to manage a department effectively, teach a client a new skill, lead a team meeting, or create a new program, just to name a few examples.

In addition, as occupational therapists, we have other occupational roles that provide avenues for leadership. In our community service and in roles as parent, friend, church member, or classroom instructor, we have a multitude of opportunities to apply these theoretical concepts to our lives. The authors in this text have stressed the significance of not only the application of leadership theories, but the integration of occupational therapy theoretical perspectives in order to address leadership challenges from an occupation-oriented viewpoint.

The continuing challenge to occupational therapists, as well as occupational scientists, is to strive to enhance awareness of the power of occupation for individuals, groups, and populations. This can be enhanced by our ability to strategically influence scholarship and practice through leadership on many fronts. This text is designed to support leadership endeavors in these multiple arenas. The accompanying Instructor's Manual is an additional resource that will provide activities for masters and doctoral level occupational therapy students. As we strive to meet our occupational therapy professional goals of wide recognition and global connection, it is hoped that this text will enable us to lead more effectively.

1

LEADERSHIP THEORIES

Sandra Barker Dunbar, DPA, OTR/L, FAOTA

Learning Objectives

1. Describe leadership from multiple perspectives.
2. Identify key leadership theories from business and management literature.
3. Understand the relevance of leadership theories to occupational therapy.
4. Apply leadership theories to occupational therapy perspectives.

> *Leaders are more powerful role models when they learn than when they teach.*
> —Rosabeth Moss Kanter

Leadership Defined and Described

Occupational therapists are often in informal or formal leadership roles within a variety of work and community environments. These unique opportunities are often experienced without a formal understanding of leadership theory or a methodical way of gaining leadership competency.[1] As the occupational therapy profession continues to progress, it is essential that occupational therapy students and practitioners enhance their ability to learn key leadership principles to gain and sustain key leadership roles in health care and community arenas.

Leadership has been defined in various ways throughout business and organizational behavior literature. Fleishman et al indicate as many as 65 different classifications in review of 50 years of literature.[2] Bass, a well-recognized author on the subject of leadership, also suggests many ways to categorize leadership perspectives.[3] Various conceptualizations of leadership include the following perspectives.

The *personality perspective* is related to particular traits that an individual possesses. Early theorists believed that people were born with characteristics that enabled them to be effective in getting others to accomplish a designated goal. Individuals with qualities such as strong social skills, empathy, and even a charismatic presence were considered to be born leaders.[3,4]

An opposing view to the perspective in trait theories is the *situational perspective*. Situational theories indicate an emergence of leadership based on various factors that arise within an environment. Referred to as *emergent leadership*, this occurs when situational demands create a leader among a group that will address the needs within a particular environment.[4,5] With these 2 perspectives alone, it may be easily understood how the controversy between the born leader viewpoint versus the developed leader has remained a continuous discussion in leadership scholarship. Some early authors agreed that a combination of these 2 ways of thinking is needed for effective leadership to occur. One may recognize a need to rise to the occasion in a leadership situation, but unless there are some inherent qualities that will allow the person to successfully lead, he or she will not be as successful.[6,7]

Power is often discussed in relation to leadership. There are various types of power, including power based on a position of authority and power based on personal aspects. People in positions of power such as CEOs, teachers, and ministers may use their status to influence the thoughts and behaviors of others.[5] Personal power refers to the type of authority that is granted someone based on his or her ability to meet the needs of the followers. If a leader is viewed as productive, compassionate, and competent, he or she is more likely to establish personal power than a person who is unresponsive to subordinates and lacks the necessary skills to get the job done. Individuals can use power in negative and positive ways, but if a leader can use power to benefit the common good and move toward the collective vision of a particular group, it will be the most optimal use.

Leadership in the 21st century is perceived quite differently than earlier descriptions of the sage or the individual who has all of the answers to organizational difficulties. Modern definitions and descriptions vary greatly, but some common themes arise from the most recent literature, including the attainment of a common goal, the recognition of leadership complexity, influencing the behaviors of others, and the need to create a vision.[8,9] For the purposes of this book, and to allow the reader to grasp a foundational perspective for subsequent chapters, the following definition will be used for leadership:

> *Leadership is a process that involves a significant degree of complexity through interactive and relational operations in order to meet the goals of individuals or groups.*

This definition acknowledges the multiple aspects of leadership by describing leadership as "complex." In addition, leadership requires not only interactions with subordinates, followers, and/or team members, but it also incorporates a degree of relationship building, with efforts to meet the goals of individuals or groups.

Servant Leadership

In 1977, Robert K. Greenleaf first published *Servant Leadership*, a revolutionary approach to leadership that impacted the corporate world as well as community and religious organizations. This retired AT&T executive promoted a unique way of envisioning the leader as servant rather than the authoritarian ruler of the office.[10] Although several other authors have described servant leadership, including references to Biblical foundations, Greenleaf is the more frequently cited and well-recognized author of this particular theory on leadership.[10,11]

In addition to perceiving one's leadership role as a servant, this approach calls for leaders to promote service from an organizational perspective and fill the gap in a society that is currently lacking ideals of compassion for our neighbor, ethical standards, integrity, and honest business dealings. Leading subordinates and followers into service leadership for the public good is a notable component in this particular theoretical perspective.[10]

Servant Leader Characteristics

Individuals lead in myriad ways. Servant leadership isn't something necessarily ingrained or sought after by each leader. One of the most significant aspects of a servant leader is that the individual wants to serve naturally and that serving is a priority in his or her way of being within the work setting, as well as in his or her general lifestyle. Following this, opportunities that embrace leadership will be sought or will naturally occur. A servant-first mentality is critical for authentic servant leaders.

Servant leaders will prioritize other people's needs above their own. Concern about followers' personal and professional growth is a key aspect of the servant leader. Servant leaders will question themselves regarding the impact of their leadership on the subordinate's needs and on whether they are moving toward their own goals for themselves or impacting society in helpful ways. Regular analysis of the effectiveness of the leadership strategies is a part of this approach to meet people's needs within the work environment as well as in the community.

Servant leadership is based on legitimate power, not on coercion or controlling strategies that require forced participation for the follower. Although servant leaders are persuasive, they are not dogmatic in their approach. Teamwork is emphasized in servant leadership, and the leader exhibits a caring attitude toward followers with a commitment to building community.

Servant leadership has characteristics that are common to other theoretical perspectives on leadership. The leader must still be visionary and imagine the possibilities of the group. They must instill inspiration and articulate the direction of the organization, institution, or even small group of people. Listening to others well and understanding various viewpoints is also key in this approach as it is in many other leadership perspectives.

In Greenleaf's seminal work, he describes servant leadership in a variety of environments, including institutional, business, education, church, and societal contexts.[10] Issues with existing strategies for leadership in these various arenas are discussed. Alternate approaches to leadership based on servant leadership are included in the chapter discussions to enable the reader to envision a more hopeful future for establishing ways of leading that promote public good on all levels.

Servant Leadership Applications

Since Greenleaf's original work in 1977, there has been an appreciation of servant leadership, but also critique regarding the oxymoron of "servant as leader." Critique suggests that these 2 contructs cannot coexist. However, the complementary roles continue to gain attention from contemporary authors on leadership, and there remains a need to substantiate the philosophical perspectives with empirical research.[12]

Levering and Moskowitz, in their review of top companies, indicated that the individuals in the best companies to work for in the United States practice aspects of servant leadership.[13] These included openness and fairness, a culture of trust, a team feeling that stands for something good, improving mankind, and service to others. Several leaders today acknowledge their servant leadership philosophies and seek to promote development in employees with limited promotion of self.[12]

Occupational therapy is based on principles of service and altruism. The humanism philosophy that supported the belief that individuals are capable of self-fulfillment provided a foundation for occupational therapy. The professional literature consistently exemplifies ideals that are common to servant leadership. Core values within the profession include respect for differences, fairness, dignity, empathy, and understanding.[14] Occupational therapy intervention is driven by what individuals want and need for themselves in regard to occupational performance. Many occupational therapists knowingly and unknowingly function in a servant leadership mode within their practice arenas by demonstrating compassion and skill in helping others achieve their goals as a top priority of their interactions.

Dillon describes an occupational therapist, Sister Genevieve Cummings, MA, OTR, FAOTA, as a servant leader in academic and other professional arenas.[15] Sr. Genevieve taught at the College of St. Catherine in Minnesota for 34 years. She is described as someone who did not focus attention on herself, but put the needs of others first, as is characteristic of servant leadership.[15] Sr. Genevieve was able to use a vision to promote the central values of occupational therapy in her multiple roles, including clinician and educator.

Dillon sought to understand Sr. Genevieve's leadership style through a series of interviews with former colleagues as well as friends.[15] Through qualitative analysis of the interview data, Dillon was able to identify several themes that were clearly aligned with servant leadership. The 3 themes that emerged included "enabling others," "focusing on the greater good," and "collaborative visioning."[15]

"Enabling others" was exemplified by Sr. Genevieve's ability to ensure that students learned in an optimal way in her classes. In addition, providing role modeling and mentoring was another way that she assisted faculty in accomplishing their goals.[15] "Focusing on the greater good" is central to servant leadership. Sr. Genevieve was recognized for her broader perspective of the academic environment that led her to consider institutional, not just departmental, needs. Her ability to focus away from herself was identified as something the participants noted, but they would have preferred that she share more of herself. However, consistent with servant leadership, focusing on others and their needs supersedes personal attainment and gratification.

Sr. Genevieve's example of servant leadership in Dillon's work enables us to grasp this form of leadership in the context of occupational therapy. Colleagues of hers continue to share her virtues and leadership style among occupational therapy students and practitioners today.

Situational Leadership

There are several situational approaches to leadership, but the more widely recognized one is *situational leadership.* This approach, developed by Paul Hersey and Kenneth Blanchard in the late 1960s, is based on behavioral and motivational theories that enable us to understand human nature and the interrelationship between human tendencies and the environments in which individuals work.[16,17] Every person has motives and needs that are evident in their attitudes and behaviors. External to each individual are circumstances or environments that influence the behavior of the person. These "situations" are also impacted by individuals based on people's unique needs and internal drives.

Leadership from a situational perspective involves the ability of the leader to appropriately assess the follower's needs as well as the environmental factors that influence the behavior of the follower. Due to the wide variation of follower characteristics and environmental variables that influence the follower, it is necessary to adapt to each unique situation in this approach. Unlike most other leadership theories, situational leadership creates a process that supports individuality in addressing the unique needs of each follower.

Situational Leadership Concepts and Case Applications

The basic premise of situational leadership is that the amount of guidance and support a leader gives is interconnected with the readiness level that followers demonstrate in participating in certain tasks or when attempting to achieve certain objectives. The guidance is referred to as "task behavior," and the amount of support is referred to as "relationship behavior."[17] Different degrees of task and relationship behavior are needed depending on the various situations a person is involved with, as well as their perceptions of their own needs.

The behavior that a leader engages in as perceived by a follower is referred to as "leadership style." Styles are adapted to fit the various situations. There are 4 leadership styles in situational leadership that describe the amount of task and relationship behavior that a leader will exhibit:

- *Style 1 (S1)—Telling*: The leader using this style provides a great deal of task behavior, but very little relationship behavior. For instance, Dominique, a new occupational therapy graduate in a medical facility, may need directives from her supervisor regarding documentation and general policies to clearly understand the expectations of the job. This high task behavior of the leader ensures that the occupational therapist will function within the parameters of the department. However, there may be little opportunity for 2-way communication to facilitate discussions at this point of the job experience, indicating low relationship behavior. Using this leadership style, the new employee must be told certain things in order to meet job expectations.

- *Style 2 (S2)—Selling*: The leader using this style will still provide significant amounts of task behavior, but will also provide high relationship interactions. For example, Dominique from the aforementioned example has now been employed for 6 months. She is feeling very comfortable in the setting and wants to ask about adapting some treatment space to optimize occupation-based treatment. She approaches the Rehabilitation Coordinator and sets up a meeting time, offering supportive feedback regarding her ideas and assuring the coordinator that she has the skills to promote change. This high task and relationship behavior leadership style enabled the occupational therapist to feel successful in the work setting.

- *Style 3 (S3)—Participating*: The leader using this style demonstrates a high degree of relationship behavior, but very low task behavior. Dominique has now been employed for one year. The supervisor tells Dominique how significant her contributions have been in the last year and asks for her feedback on how to ensure change is optimal with her noticeable client-centered philosophy of evaluation and treatment. She was instrumental in creating more natural contexts in the outpatient center and she has now been asked by the Rehabilitation Team to be on a sub-committee to revise the documentation in order to incorporate more occupation-oriented aspects for the initial evaluation forms.

- *Style 4 (S4)—Delegating*: The leader using this style demonstrates a low amount of task and relationship behavior. Dominique's supervisor often remarks to other employees how independent she is in her work and that she rarely meets with her regarding any concern or issue. Dominique has now been working at the rehabilitation facility for 3 years. She supervises fieldwork students and a certified occupational therapy assistant. She is also the team leader for the Stroke Team and contributes regularly to the department Journal Club. Providing the most appropriate leader style match for Dominique's abilities and skills created an opportunity for Dominique to be successful in her work setting.

Although understanding the various leadership styles is critical in situational leadership, it is just as important to assess followers in their ability to take on various work tasks and handle situations. The "readiness" of the follower relates to the degree to which an employee is not only able, but also willing, to participate in and complete certain tasks.[17] There are various readiness levels of a follower that will influence the style that a leader will select in managing and leading in a work setting.

- *Readiness level 1 (R1)*: The follower in this category exhibits a lack of ability or skill for necessary task completion. In addition, he or she is unwilling to engage in tasks and does not have the commitment needed to follow through with what is expected of him or her. For example, Justin is also a new occupational therapy graduate, but he lacks confidence in his skills since recently having to redo a Level II fieldwork. His supervisor notices that his notes are getting behind and that he isn't asking for help.

- *Readiness level 2 (R2)*: The follower at this readiness level is actually quite willing to participate, but doesn't have the abilities needed to complete the expected tasks. He or she is motivated, however, to make a difference and will try to improve. Justin observes a co-worker who started about the same time he did and realizes that he can do better. He starts reading his school texts more and spends his lunchtime contributing to discussions. His motivation starts to improve as he begins to get positive feedback on his contributions to discussions, and he is more willing to try to complete tasks in a timely manner.

- *Readiness level 3 (R3)*: The follower in this category has the ability to complete tasks, but lacks the willingness or sense of competence. Jennifer is a Level I student who has always made good grades in school. She picks up concepts easily and is able to critically think when posed with difficult situations. However, because learning has come easy for her, it is difficult for her to demonstrate effort in the clinical setting. She has remarked to employees that she doesn't really have to do all of the tasks because she knows that she'll pass. Jennifer exhibits strong abilities, but lacks the willingness to appropriately participate in her fieldwork experience.

- *Readiness level 4 (R4)*: At this level, a follower has the abilities and the willingness to complete expected tasks. This person is ready to perform at a high level and exhibits the confidence level to be successful in the workplace. Dominique in the leadership style section example reached level 4 in the last style example when she independently handled new tasks without direction or ongoing support. She displays a readiness for managing her tasks without the everyday supervision that a newer graduate would need.

Based on the readiness level of an individual, the leader style will adapt to meet the needs of the follower. For instance, Justin in the previous example demonstrated a need for high task behavior when he first started his employment, which corresponded with an S1 style. The leader will need to provide much guidance and direction, particularly during the first few weeks of employment for a new graduate. Matching the appropriate leadership style with the follower's readiness level will support more optimal job performance and functioning in many situations that occupational therapists are faced with in today's complex work environments.

Transformational Leadership

Burns, along with Bass and Avolio, are well known for the concepts related to *transformational leadership*.[18-21] Using transformational leadership, leaders are instrumental in creating a vision and providing the resources necessary to attain the vision through personal development.[5] The role of the leader in this approach is to focus on the follower's needs and provide appropriate role modeling for growth in particular areas that will benefit the person as well as the organization through a transformational process.

Transformational leadership has 4 behavioral components, including idealized influence, inspirational motivation, intellectual stimulation, and individualized consideration.[20] It involves a significant amount of influence that encourages the follower to achieve above-average accomplishments.[5] Followers are inspired to act exceptionally through individual interactions or through the leader's systematic analysis and intervention on an organizational level. Intellectual stimulation is the ability of the leader to foster independent, creative, and innovative thinking of the follower. In transformational leadership, the leader connects directly with individuals, focusing his or her attention on the values and desires of the follower. This individual consideration impacts the whole organizational life, and the leader accomplishes the vision by identifying key needs of various followers.

Burns distinguished transformational leadership from *transactional leadership*, which is when the leader has a different approach to meeting individual or organizational goals.[18] In transactional leadership, there is a process of exchange of one thing for another. A transactional leader will clarify expectations and how to achieve them by designating a reward for achieving the stated tasks. The leader also employs corrective measures if an individual does not meet stated goals.[18]

Transactional leadership is evident in academic and clinical experiences for an occupational therapy student. A course instructor makes expectations clear in verbal and written instructions at the beginning of a course in the syllabus. Students understand the expectations and proceed in fulfilling their responsibilities for the course. They are rewarded with a course grade. In addition, certain facility policies and procedures must be understood while on fieldwork, as well as minimum performance standards met, for successful completion of fieldwork. If criteria are not met, corrective procedures will be enforced, which may even include doing another fieldwork experience to ensure that minimal standards are met. These transactional methods are common in the development of occupational therapy professionals.

Bass and Avolio saw a need to move beyond more traditional transactional approaches to leadership and further developed the transformational aspect.[21] In contrast to transactional leadership, transformational approaches attend to the needs and motives of followers and enable them to fully meet their potential through effective and collaborative interactions.[5]

Transformational Theory Applications

There is a paucity of leadership literature in the occupational therapy profession, but an American Occupational Therapy Association (AOTA) continuing education article by Reiss provided a summary of key theories and some application within the occupational therapy profession.[22] Reiss referred to a previous study in 1995 conducted to evaluate the leadership style and organizational effectiveness of professional and technical program directors, as well as clinic administrators in occupational therapy.

Leadership style in this study included descriptions of transformational and transactional factors. The transformational factors included idealized influence, inspirational motivation, intellectual stimulation, and individualized consideration.[22] Using a leadership scale, occupational therapy assistant program directors and clinic administrators scored significantly higher on transformational traits than professional program directors did. There was a significant negative correlation between transactional leadership traits and effectiveness within the organization. Program directors with less experience indicated significantly higher scores on transformational traits, which included behavior and intellectual stimulation.[22]

Transformational leadership is evident among occupational therapy leaders who consistently create a vision and work with individuals to achieve their potential. It will be very beneficial to the profession to continue to evaluate the leadership styles and effectiveness of leaders in authoritative roles, as well as potential leaders within academic programs and clinical arenas. As we move toward achieving our goals as a profession, it is imperative that leadership development and evaluation be considered.

Path-Goal Theory

The *path-goal theory* emphasizes the accomplishment of follower goals through the motivational efforts of the leader. House, Georgopolous et al, Evans, and Dessler are among the best-known authors of this theory.[23-26] The path-goal theory is based on the premise that employees need to be motivated in order to perform well and experience job satisfaction. In addition, considerations need to be made regarding the specific work task, the structure of the task, and how this influences an employee's overall motivation.[4]

In the situational approaches discussed earlier in the chapter, the leader takes an adaptive approach and shifts his or her style based on the readiness aspects of the follower. The path-goal theory recognizes the style of the leader and the follower as well as environmental factors, but focuses the attention on what motivates the employee. The leader's role is to provide the incentives or means for the employee's path to be clear to reach his or her goal.[23] This is why path-goal theory is considered one of the exchange theories in which something may be gained from an interaction between the leader and subordinate. The leader offers something and, in exchange, the follower produces something.[24] Barriers that limit an individual's goal attainment are analyzed and removed so that the employee can more easily move forward to accomplish tasks in the work environment.

There are 4 main leadership behaviors in the path-goal theory. They include directive, supportive, participative, and achievement-oriented.[27] Each of these is stated to have a particular impact on the motivation of an employee or follower, but the influence will depend on the characteristics of that follower. The directive approach is as its name suggests and entails just telling a subordinate, with specific parameters, what they need to do. Supportive leadership in this theory is characterized by a friendly and respectful approach to employees, even to the point of considering followers equal to management. Participative leadership goes another step and invites the followers to actually be a part of key decisions within the work environment. Achievement-oriented leadership is described as a style that promotes optimal performance of followers through appropriate high-level challenges and high expectations.[27]

In path-goal theory, any of the leadership styles may be used with a variety of individuals. A leader needs to assess what is limiting an employee from achieving his or her goals and remaining motivated, then implement strategies using the most appropriate style to remove the barriers or provide motivators to enable the employee to perform better and experience job satisfaction.

Similar to situational theory, path-goal theory suggests a need to understand subordinate characteristics and consider styles that match the subordinate's needs. For instance, if a worker is unsure of his or her tasks and when to do them, a more directive approach will be successful for him or her to achieve his or her goals. He or she needs to know the structure of the tasks and expectations in order to have his or her path unblocked. Again, however, the focus in the path-goal theory is to provide an environment that will increase an employee's motivation, job satisfaction, and performance. In path-goal approaches, the leader will only provide what is needed by the subordinate, including motivational level, environmental factors, and the specifics regarding the tasks.

Path-Goal Theory Application

Occupational therapists will be able to relate to the specific aspects of the path-goal theory given our familiarity with the Person-Environment-Occupation (PEO) perspective. The PEO model[28] describes the transactional relationships between person, occupation, and environment; outlines major concepts and assumptions; and applies these ideas to an occupational therapy practice situation. The model recognizes and celebrates the complexity of performance of occupations within different environmental contexts. Occupational performance is a result of an optimal fit between the person, his or her occupation, and his or her environment.[28]

In path-goal theory, the "path" may be parallel to occupational performance. Barriers to performance in everyday functions are analyzed by an occupational therapist, similar to a leader trying to decipher what prevents satisfaction and motivation in an employee. The "tasks" in path-goal theory may be related to the specific occupations one must engage in for fulfillment and productivity. An analysis of these parts will lead to a plan that will enable a person to be more successful. This "plan" in path-goal may be likened to a treatment plan that requires a variety of therapist styles to reach certain goals. At times, the occupational therapist will have to incorporate incentives, remove barriers, or even provide clearer instructions in order for the client to reach success. This comparison to our familiar theoretical roots may assist us in recognizing key points in leadership that are feasible for application in various environments.

Case Example

Lamonte is an experienced occupational therapist who has worked in hospitals and home health settings for over 15 years. He has recently changed jobs and is assisting you in creating a nonprofit organization to work with troubled teens. You have led out in many community-oriented projects that were privately funded in the past and enjoy leading change in nontraditional approaches. You notice that Lamonte is getting discouraged after a month of this work. He seems frustrated when he is talking to other community organizers and he is far less enthusiastic than when you hired him. You decide to speak with Lamonte about his overall motivation for this type of work. Lamonte identifies that he's unsure of his role because he is more familiar with hospital and home-care intervention structure. He's not sure how to reach his weekly goals of community contacts and feels unsure that helping troubled teens is what he'll be good at, even though it's what he desires.

As the leader in this situation, you decide to blend approaches. You provide a supportive leadership style with a friendly tone and a reminder that you are partners in making this work. Then you create a written work plan with specific outlined tasks, including the deadlines for accomplishment, incorporating the more directive style. In addition, you describe your first experiences and how talking with other nonprofit workers was helpful for establishing your role as an occupational therapist in a nontraditional setting. The latter directive approach was chosen due to Lamonte's self-identified uncertainties about his role and not really feeling that he had the necessary structure to be successful.

In this case, the leader focused on the actual barriers that prevented Lamonte from feeling motivated and successful on his path. His occupational performance was hindered by some insecurities in a new role and by not really understanding the expectations of his job. The leader provided the necessary structure and support to successfully motivate Lamonte in his tasks, as well as to achieve productivity goals.

This overview of 4 leadership theories is not exhaustive in any way. The numerous theories that are available in countless forms of literature are beneficial resources for occupational therapists in academic, clinical, and community settings, as well as for students who aspire to lead at any level of future practice. Exposing ourselves to the available literature and making appropriate applications in our work settings will enable the profession to continue to move forward in a competitive health care environment.

Reflection Activity

1. Which of the leadership theories do you feel align most closely with your philosophical views of leadership? Provide a rationale for your answer.

2. Which of the leadership theories were you most unfamiliar with? How do you think you may gain from the application of specific theoretical aspects of this or one of the other theories?

3. Explore a leadership theory that was not included in this chapter and explain some of the similarities and/or differences between that theory and one from the chapter.

4. Review the Lamonte case example and analyze various approaches based on the leadership theories.

References

1. Braveman B. *Leading and Managing Occupational Therapy Services: An Evidence-Based Approach*. Philadelphia, PA: F.A. Davis Company; 2006.

2. Fleishman EA, Mumford MD, Zaccaro SJ, Levin KY, Korotkin AL, Hein MB. Taxonomic efforts in the description of leader behavior: a synthesis and functional interpretation. *Leadership Q*. 1991;2:245-287.

3. Bass BM. *Bass & Stogdill's Handbook of Leadership: Theory, Research, and Managerial Applications*. 4th ed. New York, NY: The Free Press; 2008.

4. Bass BM. *Bass & Stogdill's Handbook of Leadership: Theory, Research, and Managerial Applications*. 3rd ed. New York, NY: The Free Press; 1990.

5. Northouse P. *Leadership: Theory and Practice*. 4th ed. Thousand Oaks, CA: Sage Publications; 2007.

6. Westburgh EM. A point of view: studies in leadership. *J Abnorm Soc Psychol*. 1931;25:418-423.

7. Case CM. Leadership and conjuncture. *Sociol Soc Res*. 1933;17:510-513.

8. Kouzes JM, Posner BZ. *A Leader's Legacy*. San Francisco, CA: John Wiley & Sons; 2006.

9. Stanford-Blair N, Dickmann MH. *Leading Coherently: Reflections From Leaders Around the World*. Thousand Oaks, CA: Sage Publications; 2005.

10. Greenleaf RK. *Servant Leadership: A Journey Into the Nature of Legitimate Power and Greatness*. Mahweh, NJ: Paulist Press; 1977.

11. Blanchard K, Hodges P. *The Servant Leaders: Transforming Your Heart, Head, Hands, & Habits*. Nashville, TN: J. Countryman; 2003.

12. Sendjaya S, Sarros JC. Servant leadership: it's origin, development, and application in organizations. *J Leadersh Organ Stud*. 2002;9:57-64.

13. Levering R, Moskowitz M. The 100 best companies to work for in America. *Fortune*. 2000;1:82-110.

14. Punwar A, Peloquin M. *Occupational Therapy: Principles and Practice*. 3rd ed. Philadelphia, PA: Lippincott Williams & Wilkins; 2000.

15. Dillon TH. Authenticity in occupational therapy leadership: a case study of a servant leader. *Am J Occup Ther*. 2001;55:441-448.

16. Hersey P, Blanchard K. *Management of Organizational Behavior: Utilizing Human Resources*. Englewood Cliffs, NJ: Prentice Hall; 1969.

17. Hersey P, Blanchard K, Johnson D. *Management of Organizational Behavior: Utilizing Human Resources*. 7th ed. Upper Saddle River, NJ: Prentice Hall; 1996.

18. Burns JM. *Leadership*. New York, NY: Harper and Row; 1978.

19. Bass BM, Avolio BJ. Transformational leadership, charisma and beyond. In: Hunt J, Baliga B, Dachler H, Schriesheim C, eds. *Emerg Leadership Vistas*. Lexington, MA: Lexington Books; 1988.

20. Bass BM, Avolio BJ. *Improving Organizational Effectiveness Through Transformational Leadership*. Thousand Oaks, CA: Sage Publications; 1994.

21. Bass BM, Avolio BJ. *Transformational Leadership Development: Manual for the Multifactor Leadership Questionnaire*. Palo Alto, CA: Consulting Psychologists Press; 1996.

22. Reiss R. Leadership theories and their implications for occupational therapy practice and education. *OT Pract Contin Educ*. 2000;5(12): CE1-CE8.

23. House RJ. A path-goal theory of leader effectiveness. *Adm Sci Q*. 1971;16:321-328.

24. Georgopoulos BS, Mahoney GM, Jones NW. A path-goal approach to productivity. *J Appl Psychol*. 1957;41:345-353.

25. Evans MG. The effects of supervisory behavior on the path-goal relationship. *Organ Behav Hum Perform*. 1970;5:277-298.

26. Dessler G. *Doctoral Dissertation: An Investigation of the Path-Goal Theory of Leadership*. Baruch College, City University of New York; 1973.

27. House RJ, Mitchell RR. Path-goal theory of leadership. *J Contemp Bus*. 1974;3:81-97.

28. Law M, Cooper B, Strong S, Stewart D, Rigby P, Letts L. The person-environment-occupation model: a transactive approach to occupational performance. *Can J Occup Ther*. 1996;63:9-23.

2

DISCOVERING THE LEADER IN YOU

Jan G. Garbarini, MA, OTR/L

Learning Objectives

1. Identify strategies for leadership development.
2. Reflect and identify personal leadership strengths and skill development areas.
3. Identify strategies to increase leadership style awareness.
4. Apply leadership principles to develop a leadership vision.
5. Explore effective characteristics of leaders.

A leader is best when people barely know he exists. When his work is done, they will say: we did it ourselves.
—Lao Tzu

Before you can inspire with emotion, you must be swamped with it yourself. Before you can move their tears, your own must flow. To convince them, you must yourself believe.
—Winston Churchill

Exploring the Desire to Become a Leader

It is commendable when an individual has a willingness to explore his or her own leadership abilities as well as aspects of leadership that need strengthening. Motivation to assess one's leadership skills through continuous self-reflection is the first step to becoming an effective leader. This introspective process requires developing a knowledge base of leadership theories, seizing opportunities for application of these theories, and developing a culture of dialogue that will promote leadership development.

This process may begin with an innate desire to become a leader, or it can be developed with the assistance of a mentor. Mentorship opportunities can lead to increased visibility, advancement, and career opportunities within and outside an organization.[1-4] Regardless of whether you are pursuing this process of your own initiative or with entry into a mentorship relationship, leadership skills can be learned and developed over time using the process of self-reflection and learning activities. Self-reflection is considered a predominant force in the learning process.[5] Reflection on professional experience is critical for learning and requires contemplation of one's impact and worth.[3] Motivation for this self-reflective process can provide the fuel necessary to achieve desired outcomes noted in a leadership plan. A realization that leadership skills can be learned will energize the motivational drive within you to embark on the self-reflective process regarding your leadership skills.

Self-Reflection as a First Step to Leadership Development

Aspects requiring self-reflection consist of the following:

- Exploration of factors prompting your desire to become a leader
- Analysis of leadership skills you presently possess[6]
- Examination of the important concept of self-authorship while uncovering your leadership style
- Exploration of ways in which you obtain knowledge,[7] and how these ways of attainment relate to your leadership style
- Creation of an environment for learning, collaborative partnerships, capacity building, and empowerment for change to occur[8]

Uncovering the leadership skills that need developing through an organized process and considering contexts of immediate, proximal, community, and societal levels are also critical aspects of self-reflection.[7,9]

The structure of this chapter will assist in your progression of self-reflective steps and learning activities to uncover the leadership skills in you. This chapter will also assist in examining experiences in which you have in fact demonstrated leadership skills, as well as those situations that are most challenging to you. The particular skills needed to handle the most challenging situations can be determined and improved, promoting your critical thinking[10] as well as promoting strategies on how to "shape an environment of partnership."[11] This shaping refers to your ability to gather the necessary information, examine the social dynamics of a situation, prioritize the components of a situation, and then develop effective and persuasive strategies that motivate the desire in others to do their best. An effective leader creates a positive environment in which others want to engage.[11,12]

At the end of this self-reflective process, you will have created a portfolio providing concrete examples of your leadership style, personal objectives, and knowledge of skills needed for leadership development. Journaling and creating a portfolio will assist in the meaning and processing of being a self-reflective thinker, actualizing strategies, and evaluating and re-evaluating leadership competencies. These completed tasks will empower you to be your own agent of change with a leadership plan that can promote change at individual, community, and societal levels.

Northouse defines leadership as "a process whereby an individual influences a group of individuals to achieve a common goal...Leadership is about seeking adaptive and constructive change."[13] Grady, in terms of the occupational therapy practitioner, defines leadership as "whenever the therapist-consumer relationship empowers a consumer to reach individual potential."[14] The occupational therapy profession has been charged with addressing services to meet societal needs that are ever-changing given the economic and political situation of the country and the world.[15] This health care environment requires that leadership skills be developed among all practitioners and supports Grady's statement that "leadership is everyone's business."[14]

Current occupational therapy experts urge practitioners to consider and address the contextual implications of services in regard to occupation more broadly at a societal and population level in order for the profession to remain viable.[15-17] The need for a broad perspective is so vital that strategies to address health and wellness at a societal and global level by integrating occupation into the educational curriculum has been stressed in numerous publications.[18-21] Addressing societal needs at pivotal times requires a practitioner's commitment to lifelong learning, which is necessary for ongoing professional development given the ever-changing problems, systems, and roles.[15,22]

For effective programs to be established and delivered, practitioners must address and integrate individual, group, and/or community values.[23] This integrative process of examining and utilizing individual, group, and/or community values is supported by the Accreditation Council on Occupational Therapy Education (ACOTE) *Standards and Interpretive Guidelines*[24] and the American Occupational Therapy Association's (AOTA) *Centennial Vision*.[25] These documents have been established to prepare entry-level therapists for community practice, as well as experienced professionals who are capable of addressing societal needs.

Leadership requires an individual to take on challenging opportunities while cultivating team member cohesiveness and critical reasoning skills, including problem-solving, decision-making, and self-reflection skills. These aspects all promote the growth and the potential to support the cause with increased visibility and desired team outcomes.[1-3] A cultivated team requires creating an environment and conditions that promote motivation within others.[11] An environment is required in which individuals are comfortable in offering their opinion and in disagreeing so all sides of a situation can be analyzed by sharing viewpoints and opinions. As cited by Kouzes and Posner, "Leadership is a dialogue, not a monologue."[6]

Use of the Five Practices of Exemplary Leadership to Engage in the Process of Self-Reflection

Kouzes and Posner determined how accomplished leaders achieve extraordinary results through case and survey analysis.[6] This analysis uncovered 5 themes of practice based on a wide range of work settings and positions:

1. Model the way

2. Inspire a shared vision

3. Challenge the process

4. Enable others to act

5. Encourage the heart

Behaviors indicative of these practices were identified as the Ten Commitments (Table 2-1).

The first, *model the way*, involves a leader illuminating and dialoguing on his or her perceived values and beliefs and gathering momentum by promoting agreement that represents members of the organization. Essential to this practice are the leader's everyday actions demonstrating these shared values.

The second practice, *inspire a shared vision*, takes the first practice a step further. An effective leader is one who gathers information central to promoting positive forces and movement toward possibilities. It is blending this information into a shared vision by determining others' needs, desires, aspirations, foresight, ideas, and images that provides momentum toward achievements and obtaining goals.

Table 2-1. The Five Practices of Exemplary Leadership and the Ten Commitments[6]	
Practice	**Commitment**
1. Model the way	1. Find your voice by clarifying your personal values. 2. Set the example by aligning actions with shared values.
2. Inspire a shared vision	3. Envision the future by imagining exciting and ennobling possibilities. 4. Enlist others in a common vision by appealing to shared aspirations.
3. Challenge the process	5. Search for opportunities by seeking innovative ways to change, grow, and improve. 6. Experiment and take risks by constantly generating small wins and learning from mistakes.
4. Enable others to act	7. Foster collaboration by promoting cooperative goals and building trust. 8. Strengthen others by sharing power and discretion.
5. Encourage the heart	9. Recognize contributions by showing appreciation for individual excellence. 10. Celebrate the values and victories by creating a spirit of community.

Adapted from *The Leadership Challenge*, 4th ed, Kouzes JM, Posner BZ. 2007. Jossey-Bass. Reproduced with permission of John Wiley & Sons, Inc.

The third practice, *challenge the process*, involves promoting an environment that welcomes risk taking, seizing opportunities, and confronting challenges that foster creative strategies for improvement. This risk taking also involves learning from the experiences encountered.

The fourth practice, *enable others to act*, involves a leader who promotes collaborative efforts by instilling confidence and trust in others that foster capabilities. This capabilities approach cultivates a sense of empowerment of the individual and shared power among team members.

The fifth practice, *encourage the heart*, involves facilitating a cohesive team that welcomes challenges by acknowledging accomplishments and celebrating the success of an individual and the team. This practice establishes a climate where the spirit is nourished and an individual's and team's desire and confidence for change lead to attained visions.

An important step to discovering the leader in you is to explore and reflect on particular situations that facilitated taking on a leadership role during typical daily routines and occupations, and in conversations with others without classifying or defining our actions as such.

Leadership roles may have occurred out of your desire to influence a situation or circumstance so a desired effect or outcome would be produced. In actuality, an environment for change was being created. The Five Practices of Exemplary Leadership[6] provide a mechanism and guideline for analyzing a situation in which leadership roles were assumed.

Reflection Activity

1. Reflect on a particular situation in which you have taken on a leadership role during a daily routine and occupation. This leadership role may have occurred within the environment of your home, at work, or in the community with friends or even strangers.

2. Utilizing Table 2-1, The Five Practices of Exemplary Leadership and the Ten Commitments,[6] write a narrative explaining how you demonstrated some of the five practices and ten commitments in this role.

Use of the Concepts of Transformative Learning to Engage in the Process of Self-Reflection

Knowledge of transformative learning provides essential concepts that can assist the individual in self-reflection to transform strengths and areas needing improvement into leadership skills.[26] Understanding transformative learning theory promotes one's understanding that leadership skills are developed over time. One must be willing to self-reflect on what we do, how we do it, and why we do it. This allows one to explore new options to reach goals. Critical self-reflection consists of[26]:

- *Content reflection*: Reflection on a description of what was said or done, and the interactions that occurred that lead to a particular outcome.

- *Process reflection*: Examination of the steps that occurred during the use of particular problem-solving strategies, and our thinking processes that promoted success or that may have hindered the process.

- *Premise reflection*: Reflection on the problem, the meaning we equate with the problem, and our association with it, asking ourselves what premises we hold when dealing with the problem.

Cranton and King interlink this critical self-reflection process to being the foundation for self-directed learning and development.[26] Examining one's beliefs and values and possible alternative ways of doing allows transformational learning to come about. These self-reflective processes create one's potential to see and determine alternatives, known as transformative learning. This is a goal needed for professional development. The reflection activity below promotes an individual's potential to determine alternative approaches. The components for critical self-reflection provide a mechanism to reflect on situations in regard to what was done, how it was done, and why it was done.

Reflection Activity

1. Refer to the narrative analysis you just completed regarding how you demonstrated The Five Practices of Exemplary Leadership when taking on a leadership role.

2. Provide a description of what was said or done and the interactions that occurred that lead to the particular outcome.

   - What were the particular problem-solving strategies and your thinking processes that promoted success, and the thinking processes that may have hindered the process?

   - What meaning did you equate with the problem, and what premises were held?

3. Describe whether there were alternatives in terms of the content, process, and premise that would allow other options to have been used for handling the situation.

Use of Occupational Therapy Models to Guide the Process of Self-Reflection for the Development of the Occupation of Leadership

As competencies increase with more experience in a specified practice area, the competencies in leadership skills also develop. Occupational therapy models such as The Person-Environment-Occupation (PEO) Model[27] and the Occupational Adaptation Model[28] are helpful to guide the self-reflection process. Integration of these models with leadership theories will promote goals and objectives for the development of a leadership plan.

An assumption of the PEO Model is that the individual is motivated and is continuously developing. Therefore, there are continuous interactive forces occurring between the person, environment, and occupation.[27] Occupation is defined as "groups of self-directed, functional tasks and activities in which a person engages over the lifespan."[27] Occupation can be related to the meaningful leadership tasks and activities that are engaged in by you and others. Your leadership skills were uncovered earlier when analyzing daily activities and tasks performed in your everyday life in which you take on leadership roles. In this model, your current leadership skills and those you wish to strengthen can be used as a basis for developing your individual competencies (person).

The PEO Model[27] is well suited to promote your self-reflection and examination of particular strengths and areas needing improvement to incorporate into your Leadership Plan. This process is similar to evaluating and developing an intervention plan for our clients. In the same light, consideration must be given to establishing an environment where growth can be nurtured. This allows for the application of strategies for successful attainment of occupational goals and competencies, as well as promoting growth in leadership. Occupational performance is defined as "the outcome of the transaction of the person, environment, and occupation," indicating the dynamic interactive relationship between them (Figure 2-1).[27] Your developmental attainment of leadership skills and competencies can be considered occupational performance when applying this model.

PEO Model and an Analysis of Leadership Skills

Based on concepts guiding self-reflection, let's revisit the PEO Model and the environment more specifically. Environment is defined as "those contexts and situations that occur outside of individuals and elicit responses from them."[27] As occupational therapy practitioners, we are well aware of an environment's potential to hinder or support occupational performance and for changes within a particular organization and/or community. Occupational therapy training provides practitioners with the necessary skills to improve processes and environments that can positively influence a work setting/community.[23] When developing a leadership plan, consider occupational goals and outcomes. Outcomes should measure positive processes related to the environment that will impact on occupational performance. Remember, an effective mentorship process allows for support, acceptance, and confirmation.[1,2]

Occupational Adaptation Model

Leadership theory is also easily blended with the OA Model. According to this model, individuals have the adaptive capacity for change, meaning the capacity to perceive the need for modifying responses.[28] Occupational adaptation is the interactive process that occurs between the individual and the environment during mastery of occupational challenges within the context of his or her occupational roles. Mastery in occupational adaptation in turn promotes the desire and ability to make adaptive changes to obtain readiness skills in other meaningful occupational activities leading to occupational competency. The individual evaluates occupational responses in a selected occupational activity, measuring

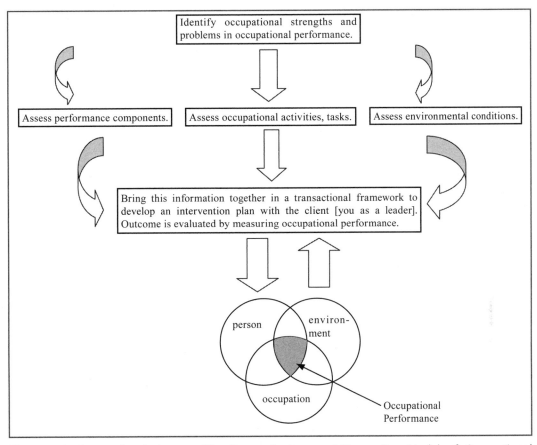

Figure 2-1. Occupational therapy: The Person-Environment-Occupation Model of Occupational Performance. Reproduced with permission from CAOT Publications ACE in Law M, Cooper S, Strong S, et al. The Person-Environment-Occupation Model: a transactive approach to occupational performance. *Can J Occup Ther.* 1996;63:9-23.

relative mastery in terms of efficiency, effectiveness, and satisfaction related to self and society.[28-30] The OA Model promotes critical thinking to enable the individual to be the agent of change.

Some concepts of the OA Model are illustrated in terms of leadership development. The therapist (mentor) facilitates the individual's (you as a leader) adaptive capacity to be the agent of change. An environment that promotes change targets the individual's (you as a leader) adaptive capacity, which promotes participation in occupational challenges (leadership skills that need improvement), facilitating adaptation and promoting occupational performance and relative mastery (related to leadership development).

As skills are developed in these leadership areas, the potential leader could strive to apply these strategies to achieve competencies also at the community and societal levels. For example, on a community level, this leader could promote listening, dialogue, and action among various community members and clients from the targeted population to facilitate their adaptive capacities to be the agents of change while creating an environment for change. These leadership actions, or occupational competencies, would result in these individuals uniting and working toward mutual agreeable goals and outcomes that facilitate participation and action to maintain health and wellness and improve quality of life for community members. These actions and outcomes address the key role practitioners can play in empowering community members to facilitate change[31,32] and to evaluate change and outcomes.[33] This key role of empowering community members to facilitate change requires an examination of environmental contexts.

It is crucial to reflect on your particular environmental contexts and the atmosphere you would like to create, consciously exploring the impact you would like to have. Explore the types of interactions necessary to create a learning environment—one that promotes inquiry, dialogue, application, and analysis of strategies and discourse to enable growth as a leader. To help you with this, let us examine these aspects more specifically in terms of reflective processes. For instance, there has been a significant change in the health care environment. A quality service delivery focus is no longer the priority in health care arenas. Currently, the focus is being placed on management-driven outcomes. It is essential for workers, as team members, to assimilate the organization's values into their delivery of services.[8,34,35] As leaders, how do occupational therapy practitioners maintain and increase the visibility of their profession's unique contribution? The value of meaningful occupations must be related to outcomes while addressing the organization's values.

Reflection Activity

1. Fill in the boxes of Figure 2-1 with your specific information gleaned from self-reflecting on the concepts of transformational learning and The Five Practices of Exemplary Leadership.

2. Examine your own occupational performance in regard to the leader in you while focusing on positive environmental conditions to support occupational performance in preparation for the development of a leadership plan. State the areas needing improvement in performance skills, occupations, and environmental conditions in terms of the outcomes desired.

3. Consider outcomes relating to cultural, physical, and social contexts, as well as personal context at individual, community (consider economic factors), and societal levels to prepare for the next section on visioning.

Use of a Vision Statement to Engage in the Self-Reflection Process

Focus will be placed on exploring your inspirations by formulating a vision statement within organizational settings. Later, we will take this a step further and examine the relationship of these leadership inspirations to competencies by integrating information from various sources, such as Kouzes and Posner,[6] Braveman,[2] and Reiss.[36]

Contextual Considerations

Since an individual's occupational performance occurs on 4 contextual levels, according to Spencer, it is imperative to examine issues of the environment that can impact on occupational performance as you strive for optimal leadership, particularly within organizational or societal structures.[9] The 4 contextual domains or levels are: *immediate, proximal, community*, and *society*. Each can have a different level of influence on participation, and each may require different approaches to promote change. As one moves on a continuum from one's immediate environment to a societal level, the amount of control the individual or advocate has on the level also transitions from direct control to becoming a participant in advocating for needed changes.[9]

Spencer draws attention to how these levels involve different processes, and that an individual's typical routine involves not only his or her immediate environment, but also engagement on community and societal levels. It can then be assumed that processes require a different set of tools and skills. There are numerous resources and strategies that assist the practitioner in examining organization-based processes and skills.[8,37] Knowledge of these processes will assist in reflecting on present leadership skills and those you wish to improve upon for leadership in a broader social context. Creating a leadership vision must integrate these contextual considerations.

Occupational therapists need to keep certain philosophical and practice aspects in mind when considering the development of vision statements within work settings. Participation enablement for the clients we serve as noted in the *International Classification of Functioning, Disability and Health* (ICF)[38] and the *Occupational Therapy Practice Framework*[39,40] are key aspects for consideration. Occupational therapy practitioners are skilled at tapping into individuals' meaningful occupations, indicative of their self-satisfaction, autonomy, and self-determination. Developing the leadership skills that enable sharing the value of occupational therapy services is what will make practitioners unique and effective partners on community and society levels. Essentially, while practitioners may treat patients individually, their role is also to be knowledgeable and a part of the larger picture within the community striving for the betterment of the public good. Organizational and program vision statements can reflect this through the leadership of occupational therapists.

Vision statements identify what you view over the horizon of time. They capture what you imagine for the future and are big picture ideas for your personal or professional arenas.[6] This clear image of what is ahead is a driving force in the present and helps to direct your actions toward productive goals. Examples include envisioning peaceful cohabitation of multicultural groups or access to healthcare for all who are in need. On a personal level, it could mean having children who will one day contribute to society and participate in helping communities build and grow.

Case Example

A practitioner works as a research coordinator in a college occupational therapy program. A vision statement was to be created that would reflect research projects focused on meaningful occupation while promoting the occupational therapy program, college, students, and clinicians in the community, as well as promoting academic excellence, leadership, and service. The vision statement was to inspire shared visions and images, promoting community partnerships and actions. Since all students and faculty, as well as some clinicians in the community, are engaged in research, this vision statement needed to appeal to all of its stakeholders. The program wanted to facilitate occupation-based research in order to lay the foundation for and empower participants with the knowledge to contribute to social justice and policy changes, fostering health promotion and wellness with the community on all levels. The research coordinator reflected on the past and the aspects that the program and community wished to achieve. These desired achievements included making a difference to the community, the pursuit of scholarly activities, improved competency in all stakeholders' occupational role performance, as well as creating learning environments that would be challenging, yet supportive and rewarding.

A vision statement was developed stating, "Through community partnerships, the occupational therapy department and community will move to the forefront, producing occupation-based research supporting engagement in occupation health and wellness."

Reflection Activity

1. Respond to the question: Why do you want to become a leader? Think in terms of a broader context, listing 3 reasons each for an individual level, community level, and societal/global level.

2. Create a vision statement giving consideration to the contextual levels: individual, community, and societal levels, as well as reflective of the purpose of the ICF[38] and the *Occupational Therapy Practice Framework*.[40]

3. If your vision statement does not reflect these aspects, keep reworking it until these aspects are reflected. This takes some time to perfect.

Strategies to Explore and Increase Awareness of Your Leadership Styles

This section focuses on an exploratory exercise that will assist you in pinpointing leadership qualities you would like to develop or refine. Two strategies that can be used to assist you include:

1. assessing your own leadership effectiveness
2. reflecting on individuals you perceive to be effective leaders

Assessing Your Leadership Effectiveness

Trott and Windsor developed a Leadership Effectiveness Survey as a tool to obtain subordinates' perceptions, and to provide feedback to the leader.[35] Leadership theories were presented in depth in Chapter 1. The development of the Trott and Windsor survey was based on the transformational leadership theory and 11 characteristics of effective leaders. Transformational leadership focuses on human relations and values, raising the level of consciousness by the creation of dialogue and shared vision (vision statement) to facilitate a follower's performance beyond expectations. This transformational leadership process also facilitates the organization's movement toward this new vision, transcending needs. The leader is viewed as an agent of change.[13]

The Leadership Effectiveness Survey[35] was adapted by this author to serve as a tool to assist you in determining whether you have tendencies toward effective characteristics of leadership and, more importantly, to provide you with an opportunity to self-reflect. The effective characteristics represented in this survey include being:

- available
- inclusive
- humorous
- fair
- consistent
- decisive
- humble
- objective
- tough
- effective
- coach

Reflection Activity

1. Complete the adapted version of the Leadership Effectiveness Survey (see next page).[35]
2. Develop a list of characteristics that are strengths and a needs list in preparation for developing a leadership plan based on findings from completing the Leadership Effectiveness Survey.[35]

Adaptation of the Leadership Effectiveness Survey

Please score your tendencies for the following characteristics. The scale is as follows: strongly agree, agree, neutral, disagree, strongly disagree, not applicable. Place an X in the box that corresponds to your answer.

Characteristic	Strongly Agree	Agree	Neutral	Disagree	Strongly Disagree	N/A
1. Available						
a) I assist others in solving problems in a timely manner.						
b) I expect that I will identify solutions, not only problems.						
2. Inclusive						
a) I readily share information with my co-workers or peers regarding organizational or school interest.						
b) I readily share information with my co-workers or peers that may be of professional interest.						
3. Humorous						
a) I have a sense of humor.						
4. Fair						
a) I give credit where credit is due.						
b) I hold everyone to the same standards of practice or academic ethics.						
5. Consistent						
a) I address issues across the board with everyone.						
6. Decisive						
a) I am determined to address issues.						
b) I am determined to set standards that impact patient care.						
7. Humble						
a) I admit when I am wrong or do not know the answer.						
8. Objective						
a) I am able to address both sides of an issue.						
b) When conflict arises, I am able to promote a win/win situation.						
9. Tough						
a) I am not afraid to address issues that would be easier left alone.						
10. Effective						
a) I assist others in identifying issues or mistakes.						
b) I am able to teach others to identify what they have learned or done about issues/mistakes.						
11. Coach						
a) I enjoy mentoring others for their professional growth.						
b) I enjoy providing feedback to others for their professional growth.						

3. Steps 1 and 2 will set the stage for a more in-depth self-assessment of leadership skills you currently have and those that need development. Additional resources for assessing your leadership style include:

- The Leadership Legacy Assessment: Identifying Your Instinctive Leadership Style[41]
- The Multifactor Leadership Questionnaire Rater Form (5x-Short)[42]
- The Leadership Practice Inventory (LPI)[43]
- The Leadership Challenge Workbook[44]

Reflecting on Characteristics of Effective Leaders

The second strategy to assist in pinpointing your leadership qualities will be accomplished in exploring and visualizing the effective characteristics of an impressive leader by interviewing one. This may be an individual you personally know within the occupational therapy profession or outside of the profession. By analyzing this leader's characteristics according to Kouzes and Posner's Five Practices of Exemplary Leadership and the Ten Commitments,[6] qualities and competencies you want to develop will become clearer to you.

According to Burke and DePoy, the opportunity to observe and compare/contrast dialogue with master clinicians and leaders allows the potential leader to view firsthand developmental steps leading to mastery, excellence, and leadership.[45] Findings from a study Burke and DePoy conducted based on interviews "indicated that mastery in clinical practice was dependent on the internal vision of practice and provides the motive for and goals of practice."[45] Excellence is obtained when master clinicians move their vision to public arenas and the vision is acknowledged by others. The opportunity for experiential learning and modeling from a master clinician/leader must not be underscored. This viewpoint provides the rationale for the importance of the experience gleaned from interviewing leaders who demonstrate the art of leadership.

In regard to "leadership as art," Grady states, "we grow as leaders by the extent to which we use ourselves as agents of change relevant to therapy goals, in promoting attitudinal changes concerning the capabilities of persons with disabilities, in understanding about all persons' need for meaningful involvement in occupations..."[14] Consider this statement in relation to self-learning of leadership skills as a lifelong process. Consider yourself as an agent of change, promoting a leadership environment so the necessary skills and goals for leadership can be obtained. Grady equates leadership outcomes and occupational therapy practice as a boilerplate for the advancement of leadership development as evident in her following statements[14]:

- Leadership, especially transformative leadership, releases human potential.
- Leadership balances the needs of the individual and the community.
- Leadership influences the fundamental values of the community.
- Leadership fosters a person's sense of initiative and responsibility.

In promoting an environment, an effective leader is one that "must harness and nurture that [leadership] drive, feed it, and encourage it to grow."[11] Shultz also speaks to the importance of creating an environment and conditions that promote motivation within others. As you read the case study of the interview with a leader below, reflect on the type of environment the leader promoted and the theoretical beliefs and principles underlying this leader's style and how the leader's action represented the five practices of leadership. Prior to reading the case study, complete this next reflection activity.

Reflection Activity

1. Briefly describe a leadership environment you would like to create.
2. Consider whether your leadership style promotes learning and collaborative partnerships in which to take risks in addition to an exchange of dialogue and discourse.

Case Example—Interview With a Leader

(Sister Agie, personal communication, October 1, 2006)

Selecting a Leader and Preparing for the Interview

I interviewed Sister (Sr.) Agie, campus minister of a small suburban college with a multicultural student population of varying social status. The challenging part of this 90-minute interview was processing so many rich, meaningful examples and trying not to get emotional when hearing and feeling Sr. Agie's compassion for those with whom she works. She has an incredible gift for words that illustrate her message.

To respect Sr. Agie's busy schedule, questions were forwarded in advance. Thus, the interview involved listening as Sr. Agie's inspiring contextual storytelling illuminated her leadership. "I will share my lived experience with you, demonstrating how students lead me in many ways."

Sr. Agie's background, including caring for babies, educating their parents, and creating a day care/preschool program for migrant farm workers in New York, prepared her for this job. She was selected due to her impact when delivering a service following the attack on the World Trade Center. Although I was lucky, only having to worry whether my two brothers and nephews would be returning home that day, helplessness and distress left its mark, as did accounts of their running for their lives. The campus minister's soothing voice, words, and spiritual guidance teased away some of my distress. What gave Sr. Agie this strength to lead and comfort others at such a time of crisis?

Leadership Style and Characteristics Analysis

Theoretical Perspectives

This interview provided an opportunity to learn from Sr. Agie's wisdom and her leadership style, which combines servant and transformational leadership. Servant leadership reflects social responsibilities addressing followers' needs, nurturing, caring, and enriching their lives to mitigate social injustices. Transformational leadership involves charisma, confidence in moral values, and expectations of followers, in turn fostering the development of self-efficacy and performance.[13] In addition, Sr. Agie demonstrates characteristics of honesty, being forward-looking, competency, and being inspiring, among others. These are characteristics of an exemplary leader.[6]

Sr. Agie describes her most important leadership qualities as compassionate, non-judgmental, and viewing individuals positively. She defines her skills as a gift. "I have a sense of where people are." Individuals are viewed as "good," but perhaps on the wrong journey due to extenuating circumstances. When asked of her interest in campus ministry involving college students, she was asked to describe what she would like to do in one word. Her response was "relate." Clearly, aspects of servant leadership and transformational leadership were theoretical and philosophical perspectives that influenced Sr. Agie.

Leadership Practices and Person-Environment-Occupation Analysis

Sr. Agie's office is in the hub of activity directly across from the cafeteria and the entrance to the main building. She is aware that the skillful use of environment enables her to serve others in her chosen occupation of ministry. She walks the halls at lunch time, participates at the sports events (interacting with students and their parents), and also frequents the dormitory. Her strategic campus roaming and participation in shared occupations make her accessible and available. Sr. Agie states, "You have to walk with them [students, faculty, and colleagues]." Sr. Agie is aware of the enabling power of balance among occupations for creating and strengthening the integration of relationships on multiple levels. She takes advantage of leisure and social participation occupations to build rapport, camaraderie, and trust with students, stressing the importance of having fun. "I get to know them on a light level, then they can get to know me on a deeper level."

Students begin seeking out her support. "I am with people and see the gifts in them, the good within." Belief in others contributes to the presence she exudes as soon as she walks into a setting. Sr. Agie uses her person, the environment, and occupations to "interact continually across time and space ... that increase ... their congruence," maximizing the fit to enable others' occupational performance.[27] "Constituents expect leaders to show up, to pay attention, and to participate directly in the process of getting extraordinary things done."[46]

Sr. Agie gathers up the students to plan and prepare food, getting on the college bus to make midnight runs to Manhattan delivering food to the homeless. Students insist they all huddle with the homeless, holding hands, and that Sr. Agie delivers a spiritual prayer before leaving. Sr. Agie states, "They lead me." She tells students, "You are the light in the darkness."

"This [experience] is empowerment from them. Students begin to see themselves as instruments. I am so privileged working with them." Touch and hugs are common, reflective that the core of a leader is the connection of his or her voice to their touch.[6] Sr. Agie builds shared values and reconfirms community, seizing "critical incidents" as opportunities to teach.[6] She always "hang[s] out," "listen[s] first," and "speak[s] from the heart," thus "breath[ing] life into [her] vision" and promoting shared visions.[46]

Sr. Agie uses analogies to teach virtues, pointing to a picture of a Christ figure reaching his arm out to pick up a shepherd about to fall off the edge of a cliff. She explains how the students with whom she works may be drug abusers, drug dealers, or come from abusive homes, trying to put themselves through school. These students haven't had the same opportunities as others. "The kids on the margin" are the students in need. "I want to journey with them when they are there on that cliff." To one student trying to leave an abusive relationship, she insisted that she call her versus her partner, no matter what hour of the day. Taking calls at night, Sr. Agie would state to this student, "Raise the praise, you called me instead of him, pat yourself on the back." Sr. Agie's relentless coaching for well over 2 years enabled this student to obtain her degree in nursing. Now working and happily married with 2 children, she calls Sr. Agie "my angel."

This demonstrates Kouzes & Posner's principles of Inspire a Shared Vision as well as Model the Way, as evidenced by Sr. Agie clarifying values based on personal values and aligning actions with shared values.[6] The principles of Challenge the Process and Encourage the Heart are illustrated by Sr. Agie's cultivation of a strategy of small wins, which actively make people "feel like winners." Sr. Agie fostered student hardiness by encouraging the change of former mindsets and breaking aspects into smaller tasks at the level this student could handle. The phrase "raise the praise" provided the student with meaningful recognition. Sr. Agie enables others to act, creating opportunities for human moments and interactions offering support. After witnessing a relative's suicide, a student remained outdoors alongside the body throughout the night during a Manhattan blizzard that hampered the arrival of medics. Sr. Agie encouraged the student to focus on past gains and not losses for continued strength to work toward graduation to put himself and his family in a better place. Sr. Agie is a heartfelt leader, mobilizing the "leader" in the individuals with whom she so compassionately works with. What an incredibly inspirational person and surely an astonishing leader!

Reflection Activity

1. Develop a list of a few potential leaders you would like to interview. With these leaders in mind, develop open-ended questions that will facilitate dialogue and the discovery of effective leadership qualities that make these leaders successful.

2. Conduct the interview and then write up the interview on each leader to gain their perspectives. In preparation for writing up these interviews, review Kouzes and Posner's Five Practices of Exemplary Leadership.[6]

3. Consider the effective characteristics that made the leader successful, utilizing the Five Practices of Exemplary Leadership as a guide to support your answers.

4. Reflecting on these interviews and what you have learned, list the effective leadership qualities you would like to develop, and 3 strategies to reach each characteristic.

Summary

It is a useful exercise for every practitioner to examine his or her leadership skills and potential to effectively impact client, organizational, and societal outcomes. This chapter has offered strategies for your leadership development. Strategies included self-reflection activities related to The Five Practices of Exemplary Leadership and the Ten Commitments, concepts of transformational leadership, and occupational therapy models that can guide the occupation of leadership. The development of a vision statement and examination of effective characteristics of a leader also offered ways to examine the leader in you and occupational performance skills for inclusion in a leadership plan.

We all have dreams to share, and together we can achieve them if each of us takes responsibility for our personal leadership practices with our consumers and associates...The place to start is where we are now by making leadership everyone's practice.
—Ann Grady[14]

Additional Self-Reflection Questions

Regarding your Vision Statement:
- Does it reflect the purpose of the ICF[38] and the *Occupational Therapy Practice Framework*?[40]
- Is it reflective of individuals' self-satisfaction, autonomy, and self-determination?[47]

Regarding environment:
- What type of environment do you want to create?
- Have you created an environment that motivates others to do their best?
- How would you like to be viewed as a leader?
- Will there be situations in which different types of leadership styles are required?

Regarding your leadership skills and those you desire to improve:
- Have the self-reflective processes provided insight into occupational performance skills for inclusion in a leadership plan?
- As an entry-level therapist embarking on community practice or as a seasoned professional, have you planned the leadership skills necessary for addressing societal needs within your practice arena or the profession?
- What "leadership legacy" will you be noted for?[41]

References

1. Bass BM. *Bass & Stogdill's Handbook of Leadership Theory, Research, and Managerial Applications*. New York, NY: The Free Press; 1990.
2. Braveman B. Roles and functions of managers. In: Braveman B, ed. *Leading and Managing Occupational Therapy Services: An Evidence-Based Approach*. Philadelphia, PA: F.A. Davis; 2006:109-139.
3. Robertson SC, Savio C. Mentoring as professional development. *OT Practice Online*. 2003. Available at: http://aota.org/Pubs/OTP/1997-2007/Features/2003/f-111703.aspx. Accessed April 27, 2009.

4. Schira M. Leadership: a peak and perk of professional development. *Nephrol Nurs J.* 2007;34(3):289-294. Available at: http://www. accessmylibrary.com/coms2/browse_JJ_N225. Accessed April 27, 2009.

5. American Occupational Therapy Association. AOTA professional development tool. 2003. Available at: http://www1.aota.org/pdt/ index.asp. Accessed April 27, 2009.

6. Kouzes JM, Posner BZ. *The Leadership Challenge.* 4th ed. San Francisco, CA: Jossey-Bass; 2007.

7. Baxter Magolda M. *Creating Contexts for Learning and Self-Authorship: Constructive-Developmental Pedagogy.* Nashville, TN: Vanderbilt University Press; 1999.

8. Goodspeed S. *Community Stewardship: Applying the Five Principles of Contemporary Governance.* Chicago, IL: American Hospital; 1998.

9. Spencer JC. Evaluation of performance contexts. In: Crepeau EB, Cohn ES, Boyt Schell VA, eds. *Willard & Spackman's Occupational Therapy.* 10th ed. Philadelphia, PA: Lippincott Williams & Wilkins; 2003:429-448.

10. Facione PA. Critical thinking: what it is and why it counts. *Insight Assessment.* 2006. Available at: http://www.insightassessment. com/pdf_files/what&why2006.pdf. Accessed April 27, 2009.

11. Shultz BJ. What makes a good leader? *AORN J.* 2003;78(1):9-11.

12. Gilkeson GE. *Occupational Therapy Leadership: Marketing Yourself, Your Profession, and Your Organization.* Philadelphia, PA: F.A. Davis; 1997.

13. Northhouse PG. *Leadership Theory and Practice.* 4th ed. Thousand Oaks, CA: Sage Publications; 2007.

14. Grady A. Leadership is everybody's practice. *Am J Occup Ther.* 1990;44:1065-1068.

15. Wilcock AA. Population interventions focused on health for all. In: Crepeau EB, Cohn ES, Boyt Schell VA, eds. *Willard & Spackman's Occupational Therapy.* 10th ed. Philadelphia, PA: Lippincott Williams & Wilkins; 2003:30-45.

16. Baum CM. Participation: its relationship to occupation and health. *OTJR: Occupation, Participation and Health.* 2003;23(2):46-47.

17. Neufeld PS. Enabling participation through community and population approaches. *OT Pract.* 2004;9(14):CE1-CE8.

18. Pierce D. Putting occupation to work in occupational therapy curricula. *AOTA Educ Spec Interest Sect Q.* 1999;9(3):1-4.

19. Peloquin S. Confluence: moving forward with affective strength. *Am J Occup Ther.* 2002;56(1):148-151.

20. Wood W, Nielson C, Humphry R, Coppola S, Baranek G, Rourk J. A curricular renaissance: graduate education centered on occupation. *Am J Occup Ther.* 2000;54:586-597.

21. Whiteford G, Wilcock A. Viewpoint: centralizing occupation in occupational therapy curricula: imperative of the new millennium. *Occup Ther Int.* 2006;8(2):81-85.

22. Hinojosa J, Bowen R, Case-Smith J, Epstein CF, Moyers P, Schwope C. Standards for continuing competence for occupational therapy practitioners. *OT Practice.* 2000;5(24):CE1-CE8.

23. Moyers PA, Dale LM. *The Guide to Occupational Therapy Practice.* 2nd ed. Bethesda, MD: American Occupational Therapy Association Press; 2007.

24. American Occupational Therapy Association. Accreditation Council for Occupational Therapy Education (ACOTE) standards and interpretive guidelines. 2008. Available at: http://www.aota.org/Educate/Accredit/StandardsReview/guide/42369.aspx. Accessed April 27, 2009.

25. American Occupational Therapy Association. Centennial vision retreat. 2006. Available at: http://www.aota.org/News/Centennial/ Background/36568.aspx. Accessed January 15, 2008.

26. Cranton PA, King KP. Transformative learning as a professional development goal. *New Dir for Adult Contin Educ.* 2003;98:31-37.

27. Law M, Cooper B, Strong S, et al. The Person-Environment-Occupation Model: a transactive approach to occupational performance. *Can J Occup Ther.* 1996;63:9-23.

28. Schkade J, Schultz S. Occupational adaptation. In: Kramer P, Hinojosa J, Royeen CB. *Perspectives in Human Occupation: Participation in Life.* New York, NY: Lippincott Williams & Wilkins; 2003.

29. Schkade JK, Schultz S. Occupational adaptation: toward a holistic approach for contemporary practice, part 1. *Am J Occup Ther.* 1994;46:829-837.

30. Schkade JK, Schultz S. Occupational adaptation: toward a holistic approach for contemporary practice, part 2. *Am J Occup Ther.* 1992;46:917-925.

31. Balcazar FE, Keys CB, Suarez-Balcazar Y. Empowering Latinos with disabilities to address issues of independent living and disability rights: a capacity building approach. *J Prev Interv Community.* 2001;21(2):53-70.

32. Suarez-Balcazar Y. Empowerment and participatory evaluation of a community health intervention: implications for occupational therapy. *OTJR: Occupation, Participation and Health.* 2005;25(4):133-142.

33. Suarez-Balcazar Y, Orellana-Damacela L, Potillo N, Sharma A, Lanum M. Implementing an outcomes model in the participatory evaluation of community initiatives. *J Prev Interv Community.* 2003;26(2):5-20.

34. McCallin A. Interdisciplinary team leadership: a revisionist approach for an old problem? *J Nurs Manag.* 2003;11:364-370.

35. Trott MC, Windsor K. Leadership effectiveness: how do you measure up? *Nurs Econ.* 1999;17(3):127-130.

36. Reiss RG. AOTA continuing education article: leadership theories and their implications for occupational therapy practice and education. *OT Practice.* 2000;CE1-CE7.

37. Baum CM, Bass-Haugen J, Christiansen CH. Person-environment-occupation-performance: a model for planning interventions for individuals and organizations. In: Christiansen CH, Baum CM, eds. *Occupational Therapy Performance, Participation and Well-Being.* Thorofare, NJ: SLACK Incorporated; 2005:338-371.

38. World Health Organization. *International Classification of Functioning, Disability and Health: ICF Short Version.* Geneva, Switzerland: Author; 2001.

39. American Occuaptional Therapy Association. Occupational therapy practice framework: domain and process. *Am J Occup Ther.* 2002;56:609-639.

40. American Occupational Therapy Association. Occupational therapy practice framework: domain and process, 2nd ed. *Am J Occup Ther.* 2008;62(6):625-682.

41. Galford RM, Maruca RF. *Your Leadership Legacy: Why Looking Toward the Future Will Make You a Better Leader Today.* Boston, MA: Harvard Business School Press; 2006.

42. Bass BM. *The Multifactor Leadership Questionnaire (MLQ).* Binghamton, NY: University of New York; 1985.

43. Kouzes JM, Posner BZ. *The Leadership Practices Inventory (LPI).* San Francisco, CA: Jossey-Bass; 2001.

44. Kouzes JM, Posner BZ. *The Leadership Challenge Workbook.* San Francisco, CA: Jossey-Bass; 2003.

45. Burke J, DePoy E. An emerging view of mastery, excellence, and leadership in occupational therapy practice. *Am J Occup Ther.* 1991;45:1027-1032.

46. Kouzes JM, Posner BZ. *The Leadership Challenge.* 3rd ed. San Francisco, CA: Jossey-Bass; 2002.

47. Hemmingson H, Jonsson H. An occupational perspective on the concept of participation in the International Classification of Functioning, Disability and Health—some critical issues. *Am J Occup Ther.* 2005;59(5):569-576.

3

LEADERS AS CHANGE AGENTS IN TODAY'S HEALTH CARE ARENA

Tara Beitzel, MA, OTR/L and Laura Schmelzer, MOT, OTR/L

Learning Objectives

1. Describe traditional and emerging approaches to health care.
2. Define leaders as change agents.
3. Describe how transformational leadership theory supports occupational therapists' interest in promoting change.
4. Understand the relevance of occupational therapists' role as change agents within health care systems.
5. Describe how occupation-centered models enable change from traditional to contemporary approaches in health care.
6. Identify how an occupation-centered approach and transformational leadership style can guide the process as a change agent in a dynamic health system.

A leader is one who knows the way, goes the way, and shows the way.
—John C. Maxwell

Introduction

The pragmatic philosophy embraced by occupational therapists allows them to become progressive leaders within the health care arena. In keeping with the Centennial Vision set forth by the American Occupational Therapy Association (AOTA),[1] occupational therapists must become more involved in influencing key decisions in policymaking to empower the profession and enhance the lives of those they serve.

Unique in nature, occupational therapy offers a broad perspective that is holistic, human-istic, and occupation-centered in its approach.[2] Historically, in keeping pace with the chang-ing modes of health care delivery of service, occupational therapists have had to alter and assume many roles, including collaborator, facilitator, consultant, advocate, and leader.[3] An additional role that occupational therapists are suited for is that of change agent. As the health care system continues to evolve, it is vital that occupational therapists take proactive measures toward developing the essential skills needed to be effective leaders of change. Specifically, occupational therapists must develop a better understanding of the following:

- Current approaches being utilized within our health care system
- What it means to be a change agent and leader
- Why occupational therapists are well positioned to lead the change process
- How to induce change

This chapter will delineate the process of becoming an effective change agent and develop a discourse for promoting change within the health care arena.

Current Approaches Within the Health Care System: The Need for Change

The idea of becoming a leader within a complex health care system seems so daunting that it is difficult to know where to begin. A quick review of past and present trends not only helps establish a picture of the current context, but it can also help clarify the leadership needed to promote change.

The ever-evolving health care system of the United States is the largest service industry in the country, exceeding over 1.5 trillion dollars in costs.[4] The amount of money Americans spend on health care is third only to that of housing and food. Considering the amount of money dedicated to health care, one might conclude that the services are meeting the needs of the people. Unfortunately, this does not hold true as for several decades, the American health care system has been in turmoil.

Socioeconomic, cultural, and political influences have been instrumental in shaping what, how, and where health care professionals practice. Historically, these influences have emphasized curative medicine and medical model principles.[4] These influences are strong and permeate health care to the degree that some occupational therapists submersed within this system have strayed from the pragmatic and occupation-centered focus upon which the profession was founded.[5] This medical model approach continues to dominate the current health care culture and has often led to high costs, decreased quality of care, and limited health care access, which can negatively impact those rendering and receiving care at multiple levels.

Consumers, professionals, and policymakers are beginning to recognize that significant change is needed to re-evaluate best practice within the health care system. The occupa-tional therapy profession has been prophetically cognizant of this need for change, and for the past 20 years has been working diligently to separate itself from the medical model realigning the profession with its pragmatic roots.[6] This realignment promotes a scope of practice that not only includes remediation, but also emphasizes the need for health promotion and disability prevention.[2] Given occupational therapy's journey back to its foundational roots, the profession is well positioned to lead in improving health care for all Americans.

The current health care system relies heavily on intervention directed toward the tertia-ry level of prevention, which focuses on sustaining life and remediating illness and injury.[4] This trend is due to the application of treatment-oriented approaches that accentuate the need to treat as many clients as possible and increase profits, often at the expense of quality of care. This philosophy emphasizes the need to treat more quickly and discharge clients at a faster rate, disregarding the quality of life of those they serve. These priorities seem to favor heroic medicine over prevention without the consideration of how clients treated within this system function once they are discharged. Extreme measures for sustaining life for the terminally ill and very premature babies are examples of heroic medicine.

In contrast, preventative education and proper prenatal care aimed at decreasing premature births and diseases, classified as secondary prevention, has been underutilized.[4] Although attempts have been made to move toward infusing more secondary and primary prevention interventions into our health care system such as preventative exams for cancer and immunizations for infants, the system has yet to completely embrace this level of care.[7] Our current health care system remains reliant on interventions aimed at the tertiary level of prevention, and at times fails to recognize and utilize the available resources of preventative interventions at the secondary and primary levels.

The current emphasis on tertiary care stems from the fact that many health care providers are trained solely under the medical model, which promotes a structural view of the client.[8] This structural view promotes the idea of "fixing" the individual and compartmentalizes the client into separate body parts. This philosophy fails to acknowledge the complexities that currently surround health care and the consumers it is attempting to help.[8] Most health care professionals continue to embody and promote structuralist philosophy and practice. Occupational therapists are often classified as structuralists even though the profession was founded on pragmatic and holistic views of the individual.[8] This misperception of the scope of occupational therapy is perpetuated within the current health care culture because even if occupational therapists practice in pragmatic ways, the intricacies of the approach may become lost by those viewing the process through a structural lens, or they are devalued because the efforts do not result in remediation of injury or illness.

Occupational therapists can no longer afford to only blend into the structurally dominant landscape. Occupational therapy must embrace its holistic foundation and lead the movement toward the use of interventions aimed at the secondary and primary levels of prevention. This requires moving away from only component views, which so heavily pervade the current system, toward a culture that embraces all 3 levels of prevention. Given current challenges in the health care field, the opportunity exists for promoting change. By taking on the role of change agent, occupational therapists can promote more holistic and humanistic ways to practice.

What Is a Change Agent?

We must become the change we want to see.
—Mahatma Gandhi

Given that you have some background information on where the occupational therapy profession is positioned within the health care system and have begun to realize that as an occupational therapist, you also have a part to play, you now may be asking yourself, "How does one become a change agent?"

Leaders have historically been known for leading others into new and uncharted areas, but what does it really mean to be an agent of change or change agent? The initial step in the process is to define change agent. The term *change agent* refers to "those individuals, internal or external to the organization, who play a significant role in fostering and promoting change within organizations."[9] Within the current health care system, change is constant. Change occurs in many domains, including reimbursement, practice guidelines, policy, and regulations, which are heavily influenced by socioeconomic levels and cultural demands.

Although change can be challenging, time-consuming, costly, and exhausting for health care professionals, it is necessary for occupational therapists to be proactive and advocate for changes that most benefit their clients. In order to effectively promote change, change agents must exude certain characteristics. The primary characteristics include flexibility, openness to resistance, respect, willingness to learn, humor, humility, and critical thinking.[10]

In facilitating change, one must first have the courage to make a change and stand behind it. Individuals must also be flexible and willing to adapt throughout the change process, as well as remain open to resistance, keep an open mind, and welcome all suggestions throughout the change process.[11] Additionally, change agents require respect, a willingness to learn from those around them, humor, humility to admit when things are not going well, and critical thinking to develop new approaches when needed. As one begins to develop a greater awareness of the characteristics of effective change agents, he or she can begin the process of reinventing oneself as a leader.

Through educational and practical experiences, occupational therapists develop the knowledge and skills to create strategies that promote change. Therefore, occupational therapists must embrace this foundational knowledge and skills and direct their efforts toward change. Along with the aforementioned characteristics, one must be positive and proactive. As depicted by Harada and Hughes-Hassell, change is a journey filled with uncertainty, yet it can be immensely rewarding for all of those involved and is worth leading.[12]

Change can occur at various levels, affecting single individuals by changing their beliefs to affect larger populations through public policy changes.[13] Using an ecological perspective, McLeroy et al identified 5 levels of influence on health-related behaviors.[14] Although these levels were originally conceptualized as levels of influence on health-related behaviors and conditions, these levels can be used by change agents as a mechanism for understanding how change can impact individuals at multiple levels.

The 5 levels of influence are intrapersonal, interpersonal, institutional and organizational, community, and public policy.[14] Intrapersonal or individual includes the characteristics of an individual, including knowledge, belief, and attitudes. The interpersonal level includes families, friends, and social supports. Institutional and organizational influences are the rules, policies, and regulations that can promote and constrain change. Community factors include the norms and standards that exist among individuals and groups. Lastly, public policy influence is the local, state, and federal policies that regulate practice and actions for change.

An example of how these varying levels can be applied to change exists in a familiar story of a woman who, after losing her older sister to breast cancer, began a mission to increase public awareness of breast cancer and raise money for research to find a cure.[15] This is the story of Susan G. Komen, whose sister led the charge to make a difference for those with cancer as a promise to her dying sister. This change agent began her efforts so that individuals like her sister would have a better chance of surviving breast cancer. Today, Susan G. Komen for the Cure is the top-rated charity in the nation.

Reflection Activity

Which level(s) have been influenced by this individual change agent?

Perhaps a more familiar change to the profession of occupational therapy was facilitated by Gary Kielhofner. Kielhofner led the charge in shifting the paradigm within the profession of occupational therapy by embracing the general systems theory as a foundational framework that now guides the development of models and frames of references within the profession.[16,17] It was this shift in paradigm that supported the development of Kielhofner's model of human occupation (MOHO) that is now commonly used to guide occupational therapy practice.[18] An example of promoting change at these varying levels within the profession of occupational therapy can be found in Table 3-1.

This example illustrates that change can occur at many levels, and it can be effective and significant, impacting all those involved. However, in order to be an effective change agent within the health care system, occupational therapists must assume leadership roles. There are multiple leadership theories as discussed in Chapter 1 that provide guidance in being a change agent. The application of leadership theories has profound effects on individual and program outcomes. Therefore, care must be taken when selecting specific styles to effectively meet set outcomes.[19] In order for a leader to be effective, the context, preferred individual, and/or program outcomes as well as appropriate leadership styles must be considered. One leadership theory complimentary to the challenges faced in the health care domain is transformational leadership.

Table 3-1. Building Safer Communities for Dementia Residents

There is a growing concern within the United States regarding the increased number of older adults with dementia residing within the community. Taking on the role of change agent, occupational therapists can utilize their skills and knowledge to foster change and provide safer communities for those with dementia at each level of influence:

- **Intrapersonal**—Occupational therapists need to be proactive in providing education to "at risk" individuals diagnosed with dementia by providing individual and group seminars as vehicles for providing important health information. This will allow those clients to develop a greater understanding of the dementia process, preparing them for the transition through the different levels of dementia as well as assisting them in planning for the future (ie, finding a caregiver to provide assistance, financial implications, legal consultants).

- **Interpersonal**—At the interpersonal level, occupational therapists can be instrumental in enhancing awareness among family members about specific community agencies through which they can access needed services. Occupational therapists can also assist in the development of support groups for caregivers, families, and friends. Additionally, occupational therapists can take the lead in educating family members and caregivers in strategies for assisting their loved ones through the stages of dementia, discussing financial concerns and providing stress management techniques for their own personal well-being.

- **Institution and Community**—At the institution and community levels, occupational therapists can provide education to the employers of caregivers of clients diagnosed with dementia to increase their awareness and understanding of the dementia process and the challenges it poses for the caregivers. Once awareness has been raised, occupational therapists can work collaboratively with employers and the employed caregivers regarding the development of strategies to assist them in caring for these individuals while still maintaining work productivity, which may include developing alternative means for completing work assignments missed while caring for loved ones.

- **Policy**—At a larger level, occupational therapists can educate and vigorously lobby policymakers to increase awareness of the need for funding for the development of programming to promote safer communities for those with dementia.

Transformational Leadership Theory: Leading the Way to Change

Just as change within health care is inevitable, so is taking on a leadership role as a change agent. As an occupational therapist within the health care arena, you will need to implement change and influence those around you by working inclusively and collaboratively.[20] Discovering which leadership theory best fits the situation and your skills and abilities is an important step in determining how you will become a change agent. Transformational leadership theory is one such theory that can guide you.

A transformational leader has been described as one who articulates a vision that can be shared among subordinates. He or she seeks new opportunities and new ways of working while motivating followers to commit to change and transcend to higher levels of performance.[9,21,22] Complimentary to change agents, transformational leaders set out to empower followers and nurture them, transforming individuals throughout the change.[22] The transformational leadership model offers a broad perspective and provides a general way of thinking about how to effectively move through the process of promoting change. Although the transformational model does not have definitive steps to follow, it does offer guidance on how to initiate, develop, and implement changes, which include creating a vision, selling the vision, and transpiring the vision.

The initial step toward change is for the leader to create a vision that can be shared among subordinates.[11,21,22] A viable vision for the occupational therapy profession is to change the current cultural beliefs of the health care system toward a greater emphasis and commitment to the practice of health promotion and disability prevention. The next step involves selling the vision by promoting it among stakeholders. In the health care field, stakeholders include consumers, health professionals, insurance companies, and politicians. Selling the vision of health promotion and disability prevention can be done through education among these parties, with emphasis placed on the utilization of holistic and occupation-centered approaches to decrease costs, increase quality of care, and improve access to health care.

Once these stakeholders are committed to the vision, the leader empowers the stakeholders to embrace higher standards of moral responsibility in achieving self-actualization and implementing the vision.[21,22] This is accomplished through a process by which individuals engage with each other to raise the level of motivation by embracing higher principles and values seeking to satisfy their higher needs. Throughout this process, the leader takes charge by acting as a change agent, transforming individual stakeholders. By using transformational theory as a guide, occupational therapists can challenge the current health care structure by promoting bolder visions and empowering those within and surrounding the health care system for any aspect of needed change.

Through the process of changing others, the leaders themselves are also transformed into more experienced, flexible, and dynamic leaders, paving the way for grandeur and more effective change in the future.[22] Ultimately, it is a cycle of individual change and growth, and when these enlightened individuals work collaboratively to effect change in the health care domain, the transformations are driven by a collective and impassioned spirit, making the changes more effective, well received, and enduring. The case example below demonstrates how a transformational leadership approach could be utilized to promote change in an in-house rehabilitation center.

Case Example

A newly licensed occupational therapist is hired at an in-house rehabilitation center. Upon acclimating to her new position as a staff therapist, the occupational therapist realizes that the intervention strategies used by the rehabilitation team are heavily based on medical model principles. Having graduated from an occupational therapy program built on pragmatic and occupation-centered philosophies, the occupational therapist wants to implement these philosophies into practice. To initiate, develop, and implement these philosophies into practice, the occupational therapist must utilize a transformational leadership approach.

The occupational therapist's first step is to create a vision of a more holistic approach to intervention(s) at the rehabilitation center. This includes staff education in the benefits of occupation-centered and pragmatic approaches, which can help transform existing intervention strategies. The second step is selling this vision to the director and other staff therapists. In order to accomplish this step, the therapist sets up a meeting with the director of the rehabilitation center (an occupational therapist who has been practicing for over 30 years). During this meeting, the therapist discusses the importance of changing the team's current intervention approach and strategies to encompass more holistic and occupation-centered approaches. The director listens attentively and decides that the occupational therapist should present her ideas to the rest of the staff.

Next, the occupational therapist presents her transformational ideas to the occupational therapy staff, inspiring the team to initiate a transition from a sole medical model approach to a more holistic and occupation-centered approach. To support and sell this vision, the occupational therapist provides evidence drawn from the profession to support the efficacy of occupation-centered and holistic practice that values what is meaningful to individual clients and creates opportunities to perform in the context of real life situations. Once the team is committed to the vision, the occupational therapist provides continued support, empowering the staff to engage with each other. Additionally, this support will aim to raise their level of motivation to implement new occupation-centered strategies into practice.

By incorporating a transformational leadership approach to change, this staff therapist initiated and developed a plan that, within a 6-month time frame, resulted in implementation of a pragmatic and occupation-centered approach within this in-house rehabilitation center.

Occupational Therapy: An Untapped Resource for Becoming Change Agents and Promoting Change Within the Health Care System

In taking time to reflect and become more aware of the leadership traits it takes to become a change agent, perhaps you have begun to identify with some of these traits. You are now prepared for the next step, which is understanding why occupational therapists are well suited to take on leadership roles in promoting change within the health care system.

Occupational therapists immersed within the medical model are still well equipped to promote change within the health care system. This change can be based upon foundational and current beliefs within the occupational therapy profession, which ideally emphasizes a pragmatic and occupation-centered approach to care. Occupational therapists have a unique view of man and of health. Consequently, they ideally view the impact of disease and illness from an occupation-centered and holistic perspective that is different than other health care professionals. These views are guided by an occupation-centered and pragmatic philosophy.[23] Additionally, these views are supported by a strong practice framework[2] and various models of practice that facilitate a connection between theory and practice.[24] Having an occupation-centered and pragmatic philosophy grounded in supportive frameworks and models of practice will not be as effective for the consumer unless occupational therapists take leadership roles to help ensure that each client receives individualized and holistic health care, offering more than traditional medically oriented intervention can provide. Achieving the best care for each consumer will require more than a concerted effort at the individual level. Subsequently, the occupational therapy profession must collectively foster and promote change at all levels.

The philosophical and theoretical underpinnings of the occupational therapy profession stem from a deep belief in the power of occupation[25,26] and the view that the human is an occupational being.[27] Occupations have been defined as activities that have "unique meaning and purpose in a person's life" that contribute to the individual's identity and sense of competence, as well as influence daily routines and decision making.[2] This definition of occupation, while valuable, does not fully capture the healing and health-promoting power of occupation.

The power of occupation arises from the innate human desire to engage in purpose-driven activities that promote growth and productivity.[28] Engagement in these activities occurs within the context of the individual's environment, thereby conceiving an interdependent relationship between the person and his or her world.[29] The role of occupation within this relationship enables individuals to fulfill basic needs, adapt to environmental changes, and develop and use capabilities in order to attain and maintain health. Through the process of performing occupations to attain and maintain health, individuals achieve a sense of physical, mental, and social well-being. Therefore, the power of occupation and its connection to health is based not only on the human being's innate desire and need to "do," but also on the need to experience, to be challenged, and to grow and adapt. The strong interdependency between the person and the environment cannot be denied or ignored. Consequently, the profession of occupational therapy embraces a pragmatic view of man and of knowledge.[8] This view explicitly recognizes how the environment, biology, and society symbiotically facilitates or hinders human performance.

The pragmatic view of the human as an occupational being also directs occupational therapists to view health "not as the absence of disease, but as an encompassing, positive, dynamic state of 'well-beingness,' reflecting adaptability, a good quality of life, and satisfaction in one's own activities."[30] This view of health, as well as the view of man as an occupational being, contrasts sharply with other professionals within health care whose focus is on fixing or curing the disease or illness.[5] Knowledge regarding how to fix or cure disease or illness is undoubtedly important. However, the application of such knowledge without the consideration of other interdependent factors can result in incomplete health care services at best and, at worst, inappropriate or negligent care. Additionally, there can be economic consequences to both the client and the public when intervention does not take into account the multidimensional nature of illness or injury. Occupational therapists are uniquely equipped to initiate a paradigm shift within health care, a shift that steers intervention toward a holistic approach and keeps occupational performance, not the remediation of disease, at the forefront of care. Occupational therapists possess the skills and knowledge to initiate this shift toward a holistic approach at each of the 5 levels previously discussed.

The *Occupational Therapy Practice Framework*,[2,31] in conjunction with holistic models of practice, cannot only help occupational therapists in directing evaluations and interventions, but it can also assist others in understanding the scope of occupational therapy practice and the process of providing occupation-centered and pragmatic health care. The *Occupational Therapy Practice Framework* supports the notion that occupational therapy offers unique services that support a pragmatic and occupation-centered approach to treatment. The domain specifically states that the role of occupational therapy is to support "health and participation in life through engagement in occupation."[31] In order for this to occur, occupational therapists need to consider more than medically oriented information such as the diagnosis, prognosis, and symptoms of the disease or illness.

In fact, the *Occupational Therapy Practice Framework*[31] explicitly guides the occupational therapist to consider not only the medically oriented factors, but also the individual's habits, roles, routines, and rituals, as well as contextual influences, including social, physical, cultural, temporal, virtual, spiritual, and personal aspects. Additionally, the occupational therapist needs to consider the demands of the occupations in which the individual wants to engage the performance skills necessary to promote successful engagement. The strong domain, which demands pragmatic consideration of the interaction between all of these aspects of performance, grounds the occupational therapist in a pragmatic and occupation-centered approach and provides a mechanism for explaining the approach to others.

Case Example

An elderly woman is hospitalized for pneumonia, and rehab services are recommended so that she can gain enough strength and endurance to return home. During a team meeting, another health care professional brings forth concerns about the patient's ability to independently manage her medications due to her failure to ask for them during the scheduled lunch hour. Consequently, the team begins discussions about the possibility of a long-term care placement.

The occupational therapist, upon hearing this, does not come to the same conclusion, but instead begins to consider why the elderly woman may be having problems remembering to take her medications. Her diagnosis of pneumonia is not necessarily indicative of cognitive decline, and although she is aging, the occupational therapist is not as quick to conclude that a decline in mental function is the cause of the client's poor performance in managing her medications. The occupational therapist, trained to consider past habits and routines, encourages the team to halt discussions regarding long-term placement until further exploration into this matter can occur.

Following the meeting, the occupational therapist asks the client about previous habits and routines surrounding medication management and discovers that for the past 15 years, the client has taken her medications in the morning with her breakfast. This routine has been disrupted by the hospital's schedule and, consequently, her performance has declined. Adjustments to her medication schedule are made and the client successfully asks for and receives her medications during breakfast. She is discharged home the next day.

This is only one example of how a pragmatic and occupation-centered approach can greatly impact the quality of life for the client and help decrease the amount of resources spent on unnecessary care (24-hour care). In scenarios such as the one depicted above, occupational therapists can help clients, but they can also take advantage of opportunities to explain to the team how the practice framework directed them to further examine the situation. This extra effort can help others within health care gain a better understanding of the scope of occupational therapy and the pragmatic process infused within the profession. This example demonstrates how occupational therapists can embrace the role of change agent and become transformational leaders by challenging and empowering other health care professionals to take more holistic views of their clients in making determinations about what is hindering their areas of occupational performance.

The domain is not the only aspect of the *Occupational Therapy Practice Framework* that promotes pragmatic and occupation-centered practice. Intervention approaches identified within the practice framework promote a pragmatic and occupation-centered scope of practice that extends past the tertiary level of prevention (remediation of illness or injury).[31] Most occupational therapy prevention interventions and programs can be categorized at the secondary prevention level. However, these interventions also encompass elements at the primary and tertiary levels of prevention. Since occupational therapists are focused on improving an individual's performance, role competence, and quality of life, their approach to intervention is often a combination of remediation and modification. This combination is quite effective as it capitalizes on the client's strengths and limitations.

In addition to the *Occupational Therapy Practice Framework*, occupation-centered models of practice have been developed in order to help occupational therapists articulate why they do what they do, and why it works.[24] The developments of these occupation-centered models, which provide the link between theory and practice, have recently been implemented into traditional and emerging practice areas.[32] These occupation-centered models support the multidimensional construct of occupation as relevant to health and well-being.[18,33-35] These models are categorized by the major domain of concern addressing the person as a whole entity while centering on the 3 common themes of person, occupation, and context.[9,32] Unique in its own respect, each model places emphasis on a different aspect, and one model is not a "fit all." These occupation-centered models provide a guide for assessment, evaluation, and intervention. In order to be effective in initiating change, it is necessary to identify which models can best guide program development, design, and implementation for making interventions successful.

Keeping in alliance with the traditional medical model treatment-oriented philosophy, these models can be utilized at the remediation level. However, occupation-centered models are not limited to this tertiary level of prevention and can be effectively used in the secondary and primary levels of prevention. These models embrace the intervention approaches of health promotion, prevention, remediation, modification, and maintenance.[2,31] The variety of intervention approaches explicitly identified and explained within the *Occupational Therapy Practice Framework* and the practice models help to connect the constructs of pragmatism and occupation-centered practice to the day-to-day activities engaged in by occupational therapy. Additionally, these models not only provide a mechanism for articulating how occupation guides the everyday practice of occupational therapy, but they also offer a blueprint for developing new occupation-centered programming.[36] Consequently, elements from the transformational model, when combined with an occupation-centered philosophy, can provide a strong foundational basis for occupational therapists to promote change. The following provide specific examples of how occupational therapists assuming the role of change agent utilized occupation-centered models and interventions to develop community health promotion programs for various populations.

Current Examples of How Change Can Occur

The first example uses Kielhofner's MOHO[18] for the development of a health promotion program for adults with serious mental illness (SMI) residing within a supportive living facility.

The prevalence of those living with some sort of mental illness continues to grow, while effective programming at the secondary and primary levels of prevention is lacking.[37] To combat this issue, effective health promotion programming at these levels is needed. Such programming (based on MOHO) is being developed for the tenants of Fostoria Junction. The tenants at this facility lack daily structure and have limited opportunities for social participation, resulting in an increased risk for depression and social isolation. Providing these tenants with a way to actively participate in structured exercise programs allows them to attain a healthier physical status, increased opportunities for social participation, and a more balanced and organized mental and emotional state.

The proposed health promotion program for this population focuses on providing a structured exercise program at the Young Men's Christian Association (YMCA). This program will focus on physical exercise and social participation while creating structure within each individual's life. This program may prevent further decline in the health status of this population while working on improving their self-esteem and increasing their sense of belonging. Additionally, they may begin to learn the benefits of developing healthy habits.

The model that guides this proposed program is the MOHO. This model addresses disruption within one's occupational life by looking at one's volition, habituation, and performance capacity in daily occupations.[18] MOHO serves as a guide to determine which specific subsystem(s) should be included in each tenant's intervention plan. The evaluation is guided by questions and assessments that seek to determine why the tenants are not fully engaged in occupations. MOHO allows each person to be evaluated individually, allowing for strategies to be customized to meet his or her occupational needs. For example, one tenant may be lacking the volition or motivation to participate, while another may require assistance with establishing healthier routines to facilitate more participation in daily activities. "By evaluating each individual using a MOHO tool such as the Assessment of Occupational Functioning, the Interest Checklist, the Role Checklist, or the Volitional Questionnaire, a better understanding of a person's specific occupational needs and interests will be gained."[38]

The Fostoria Junction program will consist of exercise programs and educational sessions.[38] The development of the exercise programs will be a collaborative effort between the occupational therapist and fitness instructors. The fitness instructors at the YMCA will administer the actual exercise programs 3 times a week. In addition to the fitness program, educational sessions will be offered that consist of information regarding exercise and benefits to health and specific equipment usage. Additionally, a follow-up session to discuss potential benefits with consumers will be included.

The premise behind MOHO is based on the system of input, throughput, output, and feedback.[18] Each of these applies to the health promotion program described above. Specifically, input occurs through the education provided by the occupational therapist to the tenants regarding engaging in regular physical exercise and the importance of developing healthy habits. Throughput entails the internal process each tenant moves through while actively engaging in the exercise program. Output occurs when the tenants engage in the exercise programs offered. Feedback occurs through the experience each tenant has with the exercise program.

A second example uses the Person, Environment, and Occupation (PEO) Model to guide an aging in place program for older adults.[34]

Given the rise in the number of elderly living independently in non-institutionalized settings, aging in place has become and continues to be a prominent issue. With the number of aging adults on the rise, this problem will continue to grow. To combat this pressing problem, community-based programs must be developed and implemented to address issues that prevent successful aging in place. The purpose of the proposed program is to promote aging in place for older adults by establishing and implementing a community-based aging in place resource and skill-building program for older adults of Hancock County, Ohio.

The PEO model is chosen to guide the proposed "Functional Skills for Successful Aging in Place" program. This model uses a multifactorial approach, addressing the individual's occupational performance from multiple levels to determine where incongruence lies.[34] This broadens the scope of interventions that can be utilized. Occupational therapy intervention would begin by assessing the consumer's strengths and problem areas within his or her occupational performance that may impede his or her independence and safety within his or her home environments. According to Rigby and Letts, the underlying concept of the PEO theory is that "the occupational performance is the outcome of the transaction of the person, environment, and occupation."[39] This model discusses the importance of matching the skills of an individual to the challenges of an activity. This is relevant to the aging population as they demonstrate age-related decline in physical, cognitive, and emotional aspects.

The PEO model, as described by Law et al, provides the opportunity for the use of a vast array of occupational therapy intervention possibilities as the individual is considered in multiple ways and occupational performance is assessed at all levels toward maximizing an optimal fit between the person and environment.[34] The different levels addressed include the individual as a single entity or as part of a family or group, as well as the community in which the individual resides. The PEO model allows occupational therapists to expand their clinical approach by identifying a lack of congruency between the individual's needs and the environment. Interventions can then be aimed at addressing the interaction between the person, environment, and occupation in order to achieve the highest level of performance. Using the direct interventions of home visits within this program allows the individual to be assessed at all levels, while also allowing for appropriate recommendations, adaptations, and modifications to be made collaboratively by the consumer and the occupational therapist. Alternative methods for engaging in activities can also be tried with the consumer to provide the best fit between personal environment, daily activities, and the individual. This approach will help familiarize the consumer with adaptations and modifications that can be made to increase safety and independence with participation in desired activities. Working with the consumer within his or her personal domain and assessing the fit between environment and consumers will also ensure that the recommendations made by the occupational therapist are indeed appropriate and do work for the consumer.

Initially, the program will provide 15 to 20 older adults of Hancock County with the necessary tools, skills, and resources for them to age safely in their own home environments. The program will be expanded annually to meet the needs of more consumers. Existing programs focus on fall prevention and home safety related to falls, with intervention focusing primarily on home modifications.[40-44] The proposed "Functional Skills for Successful Aging in Place" program takes this a step further by addressing the environmental component and providing participants with the necessary skills and resources for successful aging in place.

The proposed "Functional Skills for Successful Aging in Place" program will consist of 6 to 8 educational modules that will utilize both indirect and direct interventions. Specific indirect interventions utilized by occupational therapy and additional health care constituents include educational workshops that provide pertinent information to elderly consumers, family members, and caregivers. Direct interventions will consist of 2 home visits for individual consumers to address environmental issues and determine deficit areas of occupation that the individual may be encountering.

As discussed by Rigby and Letts, personal changes along with environmental demands have an effect on engagement in occupational performance areas.[39] Disengagement in occupations can lead to weakness, isolation, and loss of mobility, increasing the risk of falls and related injuries. Therefore, it is necessary to address all aspects—person, environment, and occupations—for successful implementation of an aging in place program. This model supports the need to determine and identify the consumer roles, the environmental demands, and the occupational performance areas in which they do and do not engage. This is required to identify the necessary interventions that will optimize the PEO fit and occupational performance.[39]

The third example utilizes the Ecology of Human Performance (EHP) Model to guide a program for overweight children and their families.

Childhood obesity is an epidemic in many countries worldwide, but especially in western societies, where it is estimated that 1 in 3 children are overweight or obese.[45] These alarming statistics exist despite efforts to promote weight reduction, thus ranking childhood obesity as a significant public health concern.[46] Adverse health effects such as hypertension, insulin resistance, and diabetes mellitus, as well as psychological and quality of life issues associated with obesity, emphasize the importance of recognizing the multidimensional nature of this epidemic and developing a plan to reverse it. Therefore, the serious and widespread nature of childhood obesity demands continued attention and exploration into new approaches.

The EHP model was first articulated in 1994 by Dunn et al and postulates that "the interaction between person and the environment affects human behavior and performance, and that performance cannot be understood outside of context."[33] The major components of this conceptual model include the person (which includes one's skills, abilities, and experiences), context, tasks, and performance. An occupation-based holistic approach to intervening with overweight children and their families must capitalize on this model's diverse approach to improving performance. Using EHP as the theoretical base of this program will help ensure that each participant's skills, context, and tasks are explored in order to determine the strengths and barriers that are impeding successful transition to a healthier lifestyle.

The EHP model offers 5 alternatives for providing therapeutic intervention: establish/restore, alter, adapt, prevent, and create. The varying approaches outlined in EHP facilitate the development of a diverse intervention program capable of addressing the person, task, and environment, thereby influencing the performance range. This diversity is needed due to the complexities associated with lifestyle redesign and childhood obesity. Flexibility within the intervention is also necessary because certain children may need assistance establishing or restoring specific skills that promote a healthy lifestyle. Family members, on the other hand, may need coaching in order to help alter the context in which the child lives in order to best support the skills and abilities of the child. Prevention will certainly also play a role as childhood obesity is directly connected to multiple adverse health effects, which continue to increase as overweight children age.[47] The direction provided by the EHP model ensures that the program developed will be both pragmatic and occupation-centered.

"We Are What We Do" is a mantra that explains the basis behind a day camp called LAFF (Lively Activities for Fun and Fitness). LAFF is a lifestyle redesign program for children aged 8 to 12 who could benefit from attaining a healthier weight. The LAFF manifesto states[48]:

> *The main goal of LAFF is to help...children [who could benefit from attaining a healthier weight] structure a healthy lifestyle around meaningful occupations and increase activity levels, leading to sustained weight loss and a reduction in future health disorders. The objectives for this goal include educating children in a fun and application-based manner about the benefits of engagement (power of occupation), nutrition, and activity level; exposing children to a wide variety of healthy activities aimed at building self-esteem; promoting exploration of skills and interests; encouraging risk taking in environments that foster self-confidence; and assisting with the development of an individualized action plan outlining strategies to adopt a healthier lifestyle.*

Occupational therapy's unique perspective of health and lifestyle redesign accounts for traditional influences on childhood obesity, and it also includes the power of occupation and the consideration of context. LAFF revolves around 6 content themes, including occupation, self-efficacy, self-esteem, nutrition, activity level, and social relationships. The power of engagement is the underlying and driving mechanism of LAFF. It is through engagement that interests are explored, skills are developed, and health-promoting lifestyles emerge. It is also through engagement that self-esteem and self-efficacy are built and new visions of future identities are born.[49]

Reflection Activity

Develop insight about your leadership and change agent abilities.

1. Review the characteristics of a change agent and leadership theories.

   a. Which characteristics do you identify with? Why?

   b. Which characteristics do you need to further develop?

   c. Which leadership theory(s) best suit you? Why?

   d. Develop a leadership plan that outlines specific steps you could take to further develop your leadership characteristics and enhance your ability to utilize one of the leadership theories.

2. In small groups, discuss these answers and provide feedback to each other regarding the embodiment of leadership characteristics.

Reflection Activity

Recognize change.

1. Review the last 3 health promotion program examples.

   a. What aspects from each of these programs fall into the tertiary level, secondary level, and primary level of prevention and why?

   b. What levels of influence do you think are required to make these programs most effective?

   c. What characteristics do you think the occupational therapist as a change agent needed to develop and implement these programs?

   d. What leadership model do you think would fit best with guiding this program?

2. Discuss your responses in small groups.

Reflection Activity

Put change into action.

1. Identify a need within your community.

   a. What is a growing phenomenon that needs to be addressed?

   b. What population is underserved?

   c. What specific problems are hindering this population?

   d. What services would be most beneficial to address this concern?

   e. What occupational therapy model would best guide the development of a program to meet this need?

2. In small groups, discuss how you would initiate this idea. How would you get started, what do you need, who are the stakeholders, etc.

References

1. American Occupational Therapy Association. AOTA adopts centennial vision. 2006. Available at: http://www.aota.org/Archive/PrArchive/2006/38538.aspx. Accessed April 9, 2009.

2. American Occupational Therapy Association. Occupational therapy practice framework: domain and process. *Am J Occup Ther.* 2002;56:609-639.

3. Grady AP. Nationally speaking: leadership is everybody's practice. *Am J Occup Ther.* 1990;44:1065-1068.

4. Sultz HA, Young KM. *Health Care USA: Understanding Its Organization and Delivery.* 5th ed. Sudbury, MA: Jones and Bartlett Publishers; 2006.

5. West WL. A reaffirmed philosophy and practice of occupational therapy for the 1980s. *Am J Occup Ther.* 1984;38:15-23.

6. Friedland J. Occupational therapy and rehabilitation: an awkward alliance. *Am J Occup Ther.* 1998;52:373-380.

7. World Health Organization. Integrating prevention into health care. 2002. Available at: http://www.who.int/mediacentre/factsheets/fs172/en. Accessed April, 3, 2008.

8. Hooper B, Wood W. Pragmatism and structuralism in occupational therapy: the long conversation. *Am J Occup Ther.* 2002;56:40-50.

9. Braveman B. *Leading and Managing Occupational Therapy Services: An Evidence-Based Approach.* Philadelphia, PA: F.A. Davis Company; 2006:197-214.

10. Cohen S. Change agents bolster new practice in the work place. *Nurs Manag.* 2006;37(6):16-18.

11. Kouzes J, Posner B. *The Leadership Challenge.* 3rd ed. San Francisco, CA: Jossey-Bass; 2002.

12. Harada V, Hughes-Hassell S. Facing the reform challenge: teachers-librarians as change agents. *Teach Librar.* 2007;35(2):1-9.

13. McKenzie JF, Neiger BL, Thackeray R. *Planning, Implementing, & Evaluating Health Promotion Programs.* 5th ed. San Francisco, CA: Pearson Education, Inc; 2009:159-199.

14. McLeroy KR, Bibeau D, Steckler A, Glanz K. An ecological perspective on health promotion programs. *Health Educ Q.* 1988;15:351-377.

15. Susan G. Komen for the cure. 2008. Available at: http://ww5.komen.org/aboutUs/susanGkomensstory.html. Accessed April 9, 2009.

16. Cole MB, Tufano R. Applied systems theory in occupational therapy. In: Cole MB, Tufano R, eds. *Applied Theories in Occupational Therapy: A Practical Approach*. Thorofare, NJ: SLACK Incorporated; 2008:39-53.

17. Kielhofner G. The dynamics of human occupation. In: Kielhofner G. *Model of Human Occupation: Theory and Application*. 4th ed. Philadelphia, PA: Lippincott Williams & Wilkins; 2008:24-31.

18. Kielhofner G. *Conceptual Foundation of Occupational Therapy*. 3rd ed. Philadelphia, PA: F.A. Davis Company; 2004.

19. Cole M. *Group Dynamics in Occupational Therapy*. Thorofare, NJ: SLACK Incorporated; 2005:55-89.

20. Brown G, Esdaile SA, Ryan SE. *Becoming an Advanced Healthcare Practitioner*. Edinburgh, England: Butterworth Heinemann; 2004:1-29.

21. Avolio BJ, Bass BM. *Developing Potential Across a Full Range of Leadership: Cases on Transactional and Transformational Leadership*. Mahwah, NJ: Lawrence Erlbaum Associates, Inc; 2002.

22. Northouse PG. Transformational leadership. In: Northouse PG, ed. *Leadership: Theory and Practice*. 4th ed. Thousand Oaks, CA: Sage Publications; 2007;175-206.

23. Meyer A. The philosophy of occupational therapy. In: Cottrell RP, ed. *Perspectives for Occupation-Based Practice: Foundation and Future of Occupational Therapy*. 3rd ed. Bethesda, MD: AOTA; 1921/2005:25-34. (Reprinted from *Archives of Occupational Therapy*, Volume 1, pp. 1-10, 1922.)

24. Ludwig FM. Occupational-based and occupation-centered perspectives. In: Walker KF, Ludwig FM. eds. *Perspectives on Theory for the Practice of Occupational Therapy*. 3rd ed. Austin, TX: Pro-Ed; 2004:373-380.

25. Johnson JA. Old values, new directions: competence, adaptation, integration. *Am J Occup Ther*. 1981;35:589-598.

26. Peloquin SM. Occupational therapy service: individual and collective understandings of the founders. *Am J Occup Ther*. 1989;43:537-544.

27. Wilcock AA. *An Occupational Perspective of Health*. Thorofare, NJ: SLACK Incorporated; 2006:51-74.

28. Reilly M. Occupational therapy can be one of the great ideas of 20th century medicine, 1962 Eleanor Clark Slagle Lecture. In: Cottrell RP, ed. *Perspectives for Occupation-Based Practice: Foundation and Future of Occupational Therapy*. 3rd ed. Bethesda, MD: AOTA; 1962/2005:65-73. (Reprinted from *Am J Occup Ther*, 1962;16:1-9.)

29. Wilcock AA. A theory of the need for human occupation. In: Cottrell RP, ed. *Perspectives for Occupation-Centered Practice: Foundation and Future of Occupational Therapy*. 3rd ed. Bethesda, MD: AOTA Press; 1993/2005:331-337. (Reprinted from *Occup Sci: Australia*, 1993;1(1): pp. 17-24.)

30. Yerxa E. Health and the human spirit for occupation. *Am J Occup Ther*. 1998;52(6):412-418.

31. American Occupational Therapy Association. Occupational therapy practice framework: domain and process. 2nd ed. *Am J Occup Ther*. 2008;62:625-683.

32. Reed KL, Sanderson SN. *Concepts of Occupational Therapy*. 4th ed. Philadelphia, PA: Lippincott Williams & Wilkins; 1999.

33. Dunn W, Brown C, McGuigan A. The ecology of human performance: a framework for considering the effect of context. *Am J Occup Ther*. 1994;48(7):595-607.

34. Law M, Cooper B, Strong S, Stewart D, Rigby P, Letts L. The person-environment-occupation model: a transactive approach to occupational therapy. *Can J Occup Ther*. 1996;63(1):9-23.

35. Schkade J, Schultz S. Occupational adaptation: toward a holistic approach for contemporary practice, part 1. *Am J Occup Ther*. 1992;46:829-837.

36. Reitz SM, Scaffa M. Theoretical frameworks for community-based practice. In: Scaffa M, ed. *Occupational Therapy in Community-Based Practice Settings*. Philadelphia, PA: F.A. Davis; 2001:51-84.

37. Rebeiro KL, Day DG, Semeniuk B, O'Brien MC, Wilson B. Northern initiative for social action: an occupation-based mental health program. *Am J Occup Ther*. 2001;55:493-500.

38. Gauger E, Weber J. *Health and Wellness: Let's Get Physical*. Unpublished manuscript. 2008.

39. Rigby P, Letts L. Environment and occupational performance: theoretical considerations. In: Letts L, Rigby P, Stewart D, eds. *Using Environments to Enable Occupational Performance*. Thorofare, NJ: SLACK Incorporated; 2003:16-32.

40. Berg K, Hines M, Allen S. Wheelchair users at home: few home modifications and many injurious falls. *Am J Public Health*. 2002;92:48-53.

41. Gill TM, Williams CS, Robison JT, Tinetti ME. A population-based study of environmental hazards in the homes of older persons. *Am J Public Health*. 1999;89(4):553-557.

42. Gitlin LN, Miller KS, Boyce A. Bathroom modifications for frail elderly renters: outcomes of a community-based program. *Technol Disabil*. 1999;10:141-149.

43. Mathieson KM, Kronenfeld JJ, Keith V. Maintaining functional independence in elderly adults: the roles of health status and financial resources in predicting home modifications and use of mobility equipment. *Gerontologist*. 2002;42:24-32.

44. Stark S. Removing environmental barriers in the homes of older adults with disabilities improves occupational performance. *Occup Ther J Res*. 2004;24(1):32-40.

45. Ogden CL, Flegal KM, Carroll MD, Johnson CL. Prevalence and trends in overweight among US children and adolescents. *JAMA*. 2002;288:1728-1733.

46. Nemet D, Barkan S, Epstein Y, Friedland O, Kowen G, Eliakim A. Short- and long-term beneficial effects of combined dietary-behaviroal-physical activity intervention for the treatment of childhood obesity. *Pediatrics*. 2005;115(4):443-449.

47. Peters JC. Combating obesity: challenges and choices. *Obes Res*. 2003;11:7s-11s.

48. Schmelzer L. An occupation-based camp for healthier children: follow the journey of creating a community-based program. *OT Practice*. 2006;Sept:18-22.

49. Clark F. Occupation embedded in real life: interweaving occupational science and occupational therapy, 1993 Eleanor Clarke Slagle Lecture. *Am J Occup Ther*. 1993;47(12):1067-1078.

LEADERSHIP IN THE COMMUNITY

Marge E. Boyd, MPH, OTR/L and Tami Lawrence, MS, OTR/L

Learning Objectives

1. Understand the historical theme of community involvement within occupational therapy.

2. Recognize the critical link between community leadership and the promotion of the occupational therapy profession.

3. Recognize opportunities for community leadership.

4. Understand how occupational therapy, community, and leadership theories can support occupation-centered practice within the community.

5. Facilitate society's discovery of the value of occupation in the promotion of health, wellness, and quality of life through community leadership.

Clearly the community is a fertile environment for verifying the authenticity
of our constructs regarding the significance of occupation in the daily lives
of human beings and in the formation of society.
—Gail Fidler[1]

Introduction

The World Health Organization (WHO) introduced the healthy cities/community concept at an international conference in 1986, following a feasibility study that took place in 1985.[2] Worldwide, healthy cities/community initiatives are at various stages of development. The challenge that the the healthy cities/community concept poses for all health care workers is to engage in a process of developing health by building on the capacities of communities.[3] Occupational therapists need to position themselves to take on leadership roles as health services move even more into the community.

One important step in assisting occupational therapists to better communicate on an interdisciplinary level necessary for community involvement was the development of the *Occupational Therapy Practice Framework*.[4,5] The *Occupational Therapy Practice Framework* uses language that is congruent with the WHO *International Classification of Functioning, Disability, and Health*.[6] The importance of the *Occupational Therapy Practice Framework* is that it provides a language that places the focus on "occupation" for health and well-being while clarifying the profession's role in facilitating "engagement in occupation to support participation."[4] The *Occupational Therapy Practice Framework* also provides language that is familiar to other disciplines. Therefore, this facilitates more fluid interdisciplinary professional communication. With occupation clearly articulated as the central focus, the *Occupational Therapy Practice Framework* can guide practitioners to practice authentic occupational therapy in all areas of practice.

What Is Community?

The word *community* derives from the Latin *communitas*, meaning "common or shared." Labonte emphasizes the dynamic aspect of people sharing membership in various and diverse groups, and this concept is central to the definition of community.[7] Occupational therapists can be members of communities on many different levels, participating in social groups; schools; or cultural, religious, or spiritual communities. Some may belong to political, sport, or leisure communities as well. They are members of the occupational therapy community and the broader community of health care teams and/or academic communities. Within the occupational therapy community, a therapist is encouraged to participate and support a group of individuals with a common characteristic. An example of this support is an occupational therapist's membership and participation in the state and national occupational organizations.

Clients who receive occupational therapy services also belong to communities. Since much of their occupational performance takes place within the context of the community, it is important for occupational therapists to consider this context. The concept of healthy communities will become clearer when community theory concepts are addressed later in this chapter. However, it is important to note the direct link between occupational therapists, the community, and community health.

The Constitution of the WHO[8] delineates fundamental principles that are considered critical for safety and good relations among all nations. First among these is their definition of health. The WHO defines health as more than simply the absence of illness or disease; health encompasses the state of well-being in physical, social, and mental arenas.[8] This definition is closely aligned with the occupational therapy philosophy of wellness.

Public health involves the protection and improvement of the health of the community through organized community efforts. The public health perspective affirms the WHO's understanding of health as a "state of complete physical, mental, and social well-being, and not merely the absence of disease."[8] This public health perspective can help us to broaden our thinking in terms of shaping occupational therapy services. In addition to habilitation and rehabilitation, occupational therapists are equipped to reduce environmental barriers, enhance occupational performance, and create prevention programs to enhance participation, quality of life, and well-being. Each of these factors contributes to public health.

Grady, in her 1994 Eleanor Clarke Slagle Lecture, *Building Inclusive Community: A Challenge for Occupational Therapy*, stated, "occupational therapists have always recognized that disability was not an illness that could be cured by medicine."[9] She suggested that occupational therapists promote and support community practice despite their particular area of practice. An enhanced sense of belonging and contributing develops when participation takes place within a community setting. Law et al stated that occupational therapists have the skills to work with architects, city planners, and others to remove barriers that unnecessarily restrict participation.[10] They also proposed the usefulness of using an occupational performance approach for measurement in a community model. Occupational performance measurement offers a relevant approach for a societal issue, and its relevance is immediately established since occupation is at the center of these issues. By assessing then removing barriers to participation, the occupational therapist can facilitate individuals returning to work or caring for themselves or others so that they can contribute to society. As barriers are removed so occupational performance can improve, the therapist is contributing to the health and well-being of the individual, as well as the health status of the community. It is important for occupational therapists to note that community perspectives and involvement in this manner is not new to the profession.

Why Community Leadership?

Several occupational therapy leaders were proponents of occupational therapy community practice, recognizing the wealth of opportunity for occupational therapists in the community setting in which individuals naturally carry out their everyday occupations.[9,11-13] Some view the community as a natural extension of the treatment setting and the locus that reflects the culmination of our therapeutic efforts. Fidler stated that the single focus and identity of occupational therapy as a remedial rehab service restricted the profession's growth.[14] Fidler advocated for a shift from a short-term, one-track medical/rehabilitation orientation to the inclusion of environments in which society could benefit from the practice of authentic occupational therapy. Her future vision for occupational therapy practice included wellness and prevention as well as lifestyle counseling programs, community planning and design, institutional design, and restorative intervention.

Within the clinic, occupational therapists are encouraged to treat clients based on evidence provided by research, yet economic pressures to produce may create barriers to reviewing evidence or conducting research to advance practice. In a leadership role, an occupational therapist may be able to influence administrators or those with decision-making positions to enhance quality service and evidence-based practice, but this is not always the case. In contrast, the community offers unique and less restricted environments for practicing authentic, evidence-based, and occupation-centered practice. Since funding can come from multiple sources such as foundations, community, or church groups, the community offers a less restrictive environment for both practice and conducting research to advance theory and practice.

Examples of Community Leadership in Occupational Therapy

Occupational therapy perspectives on leadership and community health are embodied in the writings of our scholars and theorists. Familiarity with the following authors and scholars promotes a broader perspective of the range of occupational therapy practice. These ideas encourage the use of a broader lens through which to view occupational therapy's domain of practice.

- Gail Fidler: In her 1965 Eleanor Clarke Slagle Lecture, Gail Fidler emphasized the importance of professional roles, determined in part by the community being served.[13,15] Besides Fidler's active leadership in the American Occupational Therapy Association (AOTA), she served on the board of directors of the Union County Mental Health Association and its professional advisory committee. Fidler's civic involvement included participation in various groups such as the League of Women Voters, Homemakers Program, and aftercare programs.[16] The list of Fidler's professional, civic, and national achievements is broad and extensive, and the impact she had continues to influence the profession.

- Wilma B. West: Wilma B. West was a visionary leader with a reverence for history and lessons learned, enhanced with enthusiasm for building the future. In her 1967 Eleanor Clarke Slagle Lecture, *Professional Responsibility in Times of Change*, West urged occupational therapists to identify with health services, not only with medicine.[12,17] She also suggested changing our current role as therapists to that of health agents for prevention and wellness, not just rehabilitation within a medical environment. West supported the notion that occupational therapists must consider the role of socioeconomic and cultural forces in addition to biology, emphasizing our unique focus on occupation. She warned that the specialization occurring within our occupational therapy community should be perceived as a strength, yet we should not lose sight of our common goals as a unified profession. West stressed that a unified profession can impact public decisions and policy.[12,17] Consider the hard-won successes of the American Occupational Therapy Political Action Committee (AOTPAC) in attaining and extending Medicaid and Medicare coverage for occupational therapy services.[18] The work of the Sensory Processing Disorder Foundation is another example of a small group sharing a common vision working toward the inclusion of this disorder in the next *Diagnostic and Statistical Manual* (DSM-V), anticipated in 2012.[19]

- Ann P. Grady: In her 1994 Eleanor Clarke Slagle Lecture, Ann P. Grady was a strong supporter of community practice. She challenged occupational therapists to promote the interactive model despite their practice venue and to support community practice venues "where engagement in real occupation takes place."[9] Communities offer multiple venues for meeting the occupational needs of its members. For example, programs exist for adults and adolescents with developmental delays to facilitate engagement in vocational skills. These may consist of on-site practical training at a grocery store, local restaurants, bookstores, etc. Here is a clear call to shift the occupational therapy practice arena from a hospital or medically based approach to a client-centered, occupational approach, accessing and treating people where they live and work.

Occupational Therapy Skills for Building Community Leadership

In his definition of leadership, Northouse suggests that leaders must work toward achieving common goals.[20] Thus, leaders have ethical obligations to stimulate progress toward the common good for all community members, including leaders and followers. Burns stated that individual and group goals are based on the common good. He also explained that ethical leaders consider the common good in the broadest terms.[21]

- Occupational therapists assume leadership by exercising their ability to identify community needs and resources.

  o Agents of change: Who is better at assessing and addressing individual and group needs related to occupational performance than the occupational therapy practitioner? In community settings, occupational therapists act as agents of change by identifying individual and community needs and resources. As agents of change in the community, occupational therapists recognize that individuals are a part of the communities in which they live and participate. Additionally, smaller communities must interact with larger communities. Before the therapist attends to the needs of the population, these larger communities must be considered. Identifying a point where the 2 groups intersect is an important first step. Interconnections can be "physical, cultural, personal, spiritual, or temporal."[4] After these interconnections have been identified, the next step is to identify the "gatekeeper" to introduce you (often a community leader or other influential community member who will endorse your program). Key informants or community members who possess information and insights about the community must also be identified. Careful preparation and complex community analysis serves to create a better fit for your program to serve community needs. Funding for both start-up and program maintenance are enhanced when community needs are carefully considered, resources are identified, and services are well designed to meet community needs.[22] In building leadership skills and assuming community leadership roles, occupational therapists become agents of change toward the promotion of broad-based community health and wellness.

- Community leadership is driven by the art and practice of recognizing opportunities that exist within the community. Many occupational therapists work in community settings such as public schools, recreation centers, and even home health/ early intervention. Here they have opportunities to increase their visibility in the community and to assume more leadership roles. Other leadership opportunities exist through membership in other groups such as churches and professional organizations (national and state occupational therapy organizations, charities, community events, etc).

Community leadership is also driven by understanding and envisioning the links or potential links to build resources and strengthen our community capacities. Occupational science (OS) is a significant contribution to occupational therapy's knowledge base. It can be used to hone therapists' skills in recognizing the potential links. OS was founded by Elizabeth Yerxa in 1989 when the University of Southern California's doctoral program began. It has taken on interdisciplinary and international appeal as an academic discipline to study the science of occupation. What sets it apart from traditional science is its acceptance and inclusion of non-statistical and subjective methods of inquiry while maintaining its identity as a science. OS's unique foundational base lies in the practice of occupational therapy and the recognition that adaptation occurs through engagement in occupation. As occupations are embedded in the everyday beings and doings of people, they are influenced over time and by culture and context. An extended interdisciplinary pool of scientists contributing to OS can enhance occupational therapy theory and advance treatment. The further development of OS will broaden and build upon the profession's understanding of the complexities of occupation.[23] Occupational therapists have opportunities to expand their resources to strengthen individual and community capacities as long as they recognize these potential links. By occupational therapists broadly defining health and wellness and adopting a more "systems approach" to their thinking, these potential links will become more apparent.

One example in which occupational therapists broadened their definition to include health and wellness, and also collaborated with the medical community, was in the Well Elderly Study, which was published in the *Journal of the American Medical Association (JAMA)*.[24] Using theory and research from OS to strengthen occupational therapy practice, a group of occupational therapists conducted a randomized controlled trial to evaluate the effectiveness of preventative occupational therapy services specifically tailored for independent-living older adults. This study clearly established occupational therapy's effectiveness and place in preventative health. The core concepts of the occupational therapy profession framed within the Lifestyle Redesign program[25] are as follows:

- Occupation is life itself.
- Occupation can create new visions of possible selves.
- Occupation has a curative effect on physical and mental health and on a sense of life order and routine.
- Occupation has a place in preventative care.

Using this approach, the client acquires health-promoting habits and routines. In addition to this, the client gains the ability to understand and articulate the connection between maintaining these routines and maintaining health and well-being.[26]

Occupational therapists have adapted to many different health care environments over the years from our roots in mental health through the age of arts and crafts, from the Moral Treatment Era through wartime rehabilitation, and through our reconnection with occupation-centered practice toward health and wellness.[27]

The adaptability that is characteristic of most occupational therapists is key to identifying community needs and resources. Application of critical clinical thinking skills lends itself to the identification of new practice arenas on a broad level while analyzing the steps necessary to achieve this shift into a new realm.

Applied Theoretical Perspectives

In order to take the lead in the community, occupational therapists need to integrate occupational therapy theory with leadership theory. This requires a strong grasp of the basic constructs of theories from occupational therapy and leadership perspectives. Two occupational therapy theoretical models that may be considered for application to community practice are the Person-Environment-Occupation (PEO) Model[28] and the Occupational Adaptation (OA) Model.[29,30]

Person-Environment-Occupation Model

Law et al's PEO model[28] is a good fit for community practice because it recognizes the inextricable links between the person, environment, and occupation. Within this model, each construct contributes to the client's development across the lifespan. The quality of their interaction determines the quality of the client's occupational performance. While emphasizing the client or person-centered approach, the PEO model allows for flexibility in addressing any of the 3 aspects that comprise it in order to contribute to health, well-being, and quality of life. In identifying community leadership opportunities, examination of each construct (person, environment, and occupation) can help to determine where change should occur to achieve the occupational performance goal. For example, in their qualitative study of the deaf community, Murray et al found that the PEO model was useful in identifying barriers to participation in the community.[31] Using this model, the authors identified areas for leadership and advocacy to support the integration of deaf culture into the mainstream community.

Occupational Adaptation

Schkade and Schultz's OA model[29,30] also recognizes the importance of interactions among people and their occupational environments. This model helps guide occupational therapy practitioners to recognize the client as an agent of change and to foster the client's internal ability to improve health and wellness. The OA frame of reference assumes that changes occur and people adapt to these changes according to their abilities. This model further assumes that people are intrinsically motivated by their desire to participate in occupation. This is the driving force behind the adaptive process.

Leadership

Primary leadership theories are described in detail in Chapter 1. Many leadership theories complement occupational therapy practice. For example, qualities of transformational[21] or situational leadership[32] styles may lend themselves well to community leadership and occupational therapy. In particular, Kouzes and Posner's Five Practices of Exemplary Leadership,[33] also identified in Chapter 2, are closely aligned with the basic tenets of some occupational therapy theories that guide our practice. Through their examination of leadership qualities and characteristics, Kouzes and Posner discovered 5 themes that are practiced by strong leaders (Table 4-1).[33] The accompanying commitments are described in Table 2-1 on page 14.

Consider how Kouzes and Posner's leadership principle of inspire a shared vision[33] links closely with the OA assumption of intrinsic motivation (Table 4-2).[34] For example, the occupational therapist, in seeking to motivate the recalcitrant client, takes the lead by drawing upon the shared vision of the client participating in his favorite activity of cooking. Tapping into the client's intrinsic motivation to cook links directly to the shared vision of improving (the client's) health through occupation.

Table 4-1. Kouzes and Posner's Five Practices of Exemplary Leadership	
Practice	**Description**
Model the way	This suggests that leaders' actions speak louder than words. Leaders must become involved and demonstrate their commitment.
Inspire a shared vision	Leaders must have a vision of change and must be able to eloquently share that vision with others.
Challenge the process	Successful leaders use change and innovation.
Enable others to act	This practice acknowledges that successful leadership and accomplishments are not the result of a single person. Leaders foster teamwork and encourage others to exceed their own expectations.
Encourage the heart	Successful leaders know that constituents require recognition and celebration. This fosters a strong sense of community.

Adapted from Kouzes J, Posner B. *The Leadership Challenge*. 4th ed. San Francisco, CA: Jossey-Bass; 2007.

Table 4-2. Links Among Occupational and Leadership Theory Constructs for Community Leadership	
Occupational Therapy Theories	**Kouzes and Posner's Five Practices**
OA Model	• Intrinsic motivation • Inspire a shared vision • Recognition and celebration of client abilities • Enable others to act • Expectations of occupational challenge • Challenge the process
PEO Model	• Encourage the heart • Client-centered practice • Enable others to act • Maximize the "fit" among all constructs for the client

Adapted from Kouzes J, Posner B. *The Leadership Challenge*. 4th ed. San Francisco, CA: Jossey-Bass; 2007.

Important Community Theoretical Concepts for Building Community Capacity

> *Never doubt that a small group of thoughtful, committed citizens can*
> *change the world. Indeed, it is the only thing that ever has.*
> —Margaret Mead (US Anthropologist, 1901-1978)

Consider the following concepts as you review opportunities and strategies for becoming a leader in your community. In the tradition of interdisciplinary collaboration, exciting new connections are drawn in this section between occupational therapy and models from economics and social science. The relationships between each concept and occupational therapy theory are demonstrated in the examples following this introduction of key community concepts.

The Capabilities Approach[35] was introduced by Amartya Sen, winner of the 1998 Nobel Peace Prize in Economics. This is a development economics approach that distinguishes between what a person actually achieves and what a person could possibly achieve. It allows one to consider qualitative differences such as the difference between income and a life well lived.[35]

Sen proposed that quality of life should be measured by freedom as opposed to wealth. He used the term *unfreedom* to indicate a barrier to freedom and economic development. Sen viewed his Capabilities Approach as a means to convert resources and capacity into capability. In other words, it is less about the resources and more about the actual change that occurs. Are people now able to do things that they value, or to become the people they wish to be, as a result of having freer access to resources? Also, do they have the capabilities necessary to elicit this transformation to a better life?[35,36]

Parallels with occupational therapy are evident. Sen's concept of a life well lived is congruent with occupational therapy's new brand of "living life to its fullest," introduced by Penelope Moyers in her Presidential Address.[37] Moyers describes "living life to its fullest" as the essence of occupational therapy in that we help people make the impossible possible.[37] Further, the concept of occupational deprivation is similar to Sen's notion of "unfreedom." Occupational deprivation is a state in which individuals are prevented from participation in meaningful occupation due to circumstances that are beyond their control,[38] resulting in limited or no access to resources.

A number of variables are engaged in a Capabilities Approach, including personal capacity (human capital drive, impairment, resources, gender, race, and ethnicity) and commodities (individually and collectively, owned and shared), and the opportunity gradient that connects individuals to the capability set (locally valued beings and doings) and actual functionings (the choices that individuals make and the way that they actually function). The opportunity gradient, in turn, is affected by the social and cultural norms, demands, expectations, and environment (law, custom, policy, regulation, and representations) (Figure 4-1).[35]

To illustrate the concept of Sen's Capabilities Approach, consider the case of an individual who is starving. What individual "unfreedom" or, in occupational therapy terms, "barrier to occupational performance" is at the root of this starvation? Perhaps the individual is starving because he is unable to afford food. The individual may be in a war zone where it is impossible to transport food, in a political prison where food is denied, or perhaps the person has a disability that affects swallowing. In each of these cases, the control is outside of the person, but there may be other reasons such as anorexia or religious or political fasting in which the control is within the person. Each of these situations would require a different response based on the quality of the situation and the unfreedoms that apply. Now reconsider the parallels between Sen's model and the concept of occupational deprivation.

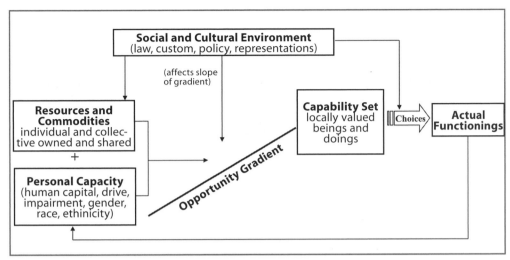

Figure 4-1. Converting resources and capacity into capabilities: Sen's Capabilities Approach. Designed by Dr. K. Hopper, Nathan Kline Institute for Psychiatric Research and Center to Study Recovery in Social Context, Spring 2008.[35]

Such deprivation could be caused by depression and withdrawal, being an infant in a large understaffed orphanage, having a spinal cord injury, or spending time in a bomb shelter.[39]

Consider how smoothly Sen's economic philosophy translates into the language of occupational therapy. The occupational therapist seeking to help an individual achieve his or her full potential is concerned with the occupational freedom of a person (ie, a person's ability to participate in meaningful occupation). Through occupation, the individual enters a process of adaptation. Occupational therapists work with individuals who are immobilized through accidents, disease, or sometimes the aging process. This loss of movement or occupational deprivation can be regarded as an "unfreedom" or barrier to participation in meaningful occupation. This barrier to the adaptive process has implications for mental health.

A significant finding in a study by Lipowski on sensory deprivation suggests that "immobilization is the most disabling form of deprivation, and that, if added to other sensory losses, is very likely to produce psychiatric symptoms in the vulnerable."[40] Extensive research on the stress response to immobilization in both human and animal studies supports the claim that immobilization causes significant stress. Lipowski's study highlights the need for occupation-centered practice, focusing on adaptation and prevention for individuals who have experienced the occupational deprivation of immobilization.

It would be useful for occupational therapists to familiarize themselves with Sen's Capabilities Approach as this is a widely hailed economic model for addressing health and disability disparities.[35] From a leadership stance, assimilation of these concepts will strengthen the participation of occupational therapists involved in disability policy. Of course, some occupational therapists may feel that this broader application of occupational therapy is beyond their scope or preference. As a practitioner, however, it is important to be a contributor in some way to the larger system, even if it means taking a leadership role in collecting data within the clinic or community to inform the larger process.

Related Community Practice Terms

Familiarity with the following (social science) community terms is useful as we expand our understanding of occupation, participation, and the community:

- Community collaboration is the result of sharing knowledge, resulting in a revised joint understanding of this knowledge.[41] The collaborative process is critical to community work. It is the collaborative process that fosters understanding and participation among the stakeholders.

- Community capacities are the characteristics of a community and their impact on its ability to recognize problems, organize itself, and address its problems. Community capacity can be observed in community patterns, community leadership, social networks, and the community member's access to power.[42]

- Community capacity building is the process of empowering community members by way of education, networking, and participation in identifying problems, solutions to problems, and the ability to access power.[42] Rather than focusing on the needs of the community, a capabilities approach focuses on community capacities upon which members can build. This concept is closely linked to the occupational therapy perspective of emphasizing ability and function rather than disability, as well as to the PEO model, which emphasizes interactions among community, members, and tasks.

- Empowerment theory began as a social science theory in which "individuals and groups gain power, access to resources, and control over their own lives. In doing so, they gain the ability to achieve their highest personal and collective aspirations and goals."[43] This theory evolved as a response to feelings of powerlessness among people with disabilities and those who supported them. The process of empowerment involves movement through the following stages of[44]:
  1. Awareness
  2. Connecting and learning
  3. Taking action
  4. Contribution

As the individual progresses through these stages, the health care practitioner provides support and guidance as necessary. There is no final end point in this process. Instead, individuals may continuously develop awareness of deficits or needs in various domains of their lives (work, leisure, etc), creating a constantly changing role for the health care practitioner. This theory is useful for creating links between the constructs of leadership, occupation, and community. For example, occupational therapists collaborate with their clients to identify treatment objectives and seek to empower them to achieve their identified goals.

Addressing Community Needs

Occupational therapists are well aware of the mental and physical deterioration that occurs when an individual ceases to engage in meaningful occupation. Community issues such as violence, mental illness, drug and alcohol abuse, aging, and others create community problems. Within the community, occupational therapists can assist citizens to improve their health, well-being, and quality of life through changes in the environment and social policy. Today's community needs are significant, and the philosophical base addressing these issues has been developed over time.

Baum and Law referred to community health as both a responsibility and an opportunity, as well as a good fit for occupational therapy.[11] The WHO's Healthy Communities movement pushing for communities to promote healthy community environments and National Institutes of Health (NIH) support for community health initiatives is available. What better time to draw upon occupational therapy's interdisciplinary roots to lead and join initiatives to improve community health?[11] Who will heed the words of community leaders in occupational therapy, such as Adolph Meyer, Mary Reilly, Wilma West, and Gail Fidler, to bring the power of occupation into the community?

Methods for Evaluating Community Activity

Participatory action research (PAR) provides a framework in which people with disabilities can assume an active role in designing and conducting the research that will ultimately empower them to address their independent living and rehabilitation goals.[45] In PAR, the intent is that change will occur, while knowledge is generated through the process. The knowledge generated is a result of respect for different ways of knowing and close collaboration between the clients and experts who contribute to the process.[46] Taylor et al delineate the methods of PAR as the following[47]:

- Delineating the problem
- Choosing the action
- Designing and assessing research methods
- Engaging in action
- Gathering data
- Reflexive knowledge (an empowering review of the process and outcomes)

Participatory evaluation research is a powerful tool that can be useful in sustaining community commitments, empowering clients, and promoting the growth of the occupational therapy profession through disabilities research. In participatory evaluation research, the action is not the primary purpose.[46]

The 5 participatory evaluation phases are as follows[48]:

1. *Phase I*: Developing a partnership and planning the evaluation—The process of engaging in a conversation about a desired community project with citizen leaders and community members for a collaborative partnership. Mutual respect for contributions is an expectation.

2. *Phase II*: Developing a logic model—The process of brainstorming sessions about program outcomes, designed to connect the program goals, resources, activities, outputs, and specific changes in the community, taking into consideration the best evidence and determining the indicators of program success for proper documentation.

3. *Phase III*: Identifying the methodology and data collection strategies—Decisions are made about what data will be collected and by which method. Before implementing research, proposals are submitted to the Institutional Review Board for approval.

4. *Phase IV*: Interpreting and reporting findings—Community agencies attend research meetings and provide input so that changes can be implemented as needed. Some community members collect data, and researchers analyze these data.

5. *Phase V*: Feedback, monitoring, and utilization of the findings—As participants become empowered, they begin to use the information generated to help themselves and their communities.

A significant goal of PAR is the transformation of community members as they begin to understand how they can gain control of their community organizations. Community building capacities are strengthened within this process.[48]

The concept of Healthy Communities[42] illustrates PAR on a broad scale. Healthy Communities "are those that continually create and improve those physical and social environments and expand those community resources that enable people to mutually support each other in performing all of the functions of life and in developing to their maximum potential."[42] This commonly accepted definition of a healthy community was originally proposed by Hancock and Duhl for the WHO in 1993. The underlying concept here is that attaining and sustaining a "healthy community" is an ongoing process reflective of the attitudes and actions of the primary stakeholders and the members of the community.

Integrating Community Theory

The following practical examples of community leadership embody concepts of empowerment theory, community building and organizing, capacity building, Capabilities Approach, PAR, and participatory evaluation research.

The following section describes the Center for Vision Education using a Capabilities Approach.

Case Example

To illustrate concepts of community theory, consider the following college-community collaboration. The "Community Center for Visual Education," a college-based project, was created to meet a community need for low-vision education. The college education department received a grant for $75,000 to purchase equipment for individuals with low vision. The occupational therapy program was invited to be a part of the equipment selection process. Adaptive utensils, including a talking microwave, a talking coffee maker, and several high-powered reading machines, were purchased for the occupational therapy kitchen and reading room.

To better empower community members and build stronger community ties, the college chancellor decided that this project should be run by the community. The equipment company trained members of a local organization on the reading equipment, while other volunteers were recruited to transport community members who wished to use the center. Community members collaborated with the chancellor to identify members with low vision who wanted to learn about adaptations to enhance their lives. The chancellor arranged an open house in conjunction with the new health and science building.

Several community members with low vision and members of the community organization, education department, and occupational therapy faculty, as well as the chancellor, met to discuss future plans for the community-driven center. Community collaboration occurred as each stakeholder was empowered at a certain level. The chancellor was empowered to meet the educational needs of the community without having to tax limited college and faculty resources. The community organization was empowered to carry out its mission of community service while gaining new skills, and the community members with low vision were empowered to learn about life-enhancing adaptations. The community organization demonstrated community capacity by organizing itself to meet the needs of the community. Other communities with limited community capacity may not have been able to organize in such an effective way.

As the Community Center for Vision Education was established, and as volunteers and community members with low vision visited the center on a more regular basis, the occupational therapy research and academic coordinators collaborated with stakeholders to develop a PAR initiative. A group of individuals with low vision met with the research and academic coordinators to create a logic plan. The research coordinator and academic coordinator determined that research students could carry out research projects in conjunction with the community organization. Research students made large-print educational and low-vision resource packets for the community members with low vision and provided them with an orientation to the adaptive utensils and equipment. The effectiveness of the orientation was measured by means of a pre- and post-test qualitative survey. The significance of the surveys was that the visitors to the center contributed to the research that would ultimately be used to benefit them and future visitors who seek to learn more about how to live well with their disability.

Using a Capabilities Approach, the project's occupational therapist played a key role in assessing the personal capacities of the center visitors, considering human capital, drive, the level of impairment, gender, race, and ethnicity.

Any of these could impact one's freedom. For instance, certain gender-related roles may have been significantly impacted by the individual's low vision. The collectively owned and shared resources and commodities allowed the grant to become a reality and the community group to organize. Because of this ability to organize, center visitors without access to transportation could be driven by volunteers and receive training on the low-vision equipment by other trained community volunteers. With the center's mission of education, the possible functionings or achievements of individual community members with low vision (or what may be expected of the individual) were compared to their actual functionings or achievements. If the person's actual functionings failed to match his or her possible functionings, or if the client did not make the expected progress based on his or her assessed potential, the therapist explored "unfreedoms" or barriers that affected the individual's capability to achieve. Using a Capabilities Approach, the therapist engaged in a broader view of factors influencing occupational performance, incorporating concepts from Capabilities Approach, public health, and WHO perspectives.

Case Example

Another illustration of these constructs in action takes place in the development of a local nonprofit foundation designed to meet a need within a specific community. A local occupational therapist working in early intervention noted that many families experienced significant delays and challenges in obtaining diagnoses and services for their young children, particularly those with possible autism spectrum diagnoses.

Further investigation revealed that although families shared concerns with their pediatricians, they were referred to a diagnostic center several hours away and put on a 6+ month waiting list for evaluation. Typically, they were unable to access insured intervention services during this waiting period.

The occupational therapist recruited a friend with experience as a community volunteer and together they drafted a plan to alleviate this need. They formed the Lowcountry Autism Foundation, Inc. The organizational mission is to provide broad support, including financial support, intervention services, and advocacy, for individuals and families who face the challenges of living with autism. Specific goals include promoting awareness that optimal developmental outcomes are achieved through the earliest possible screening and diagnosis by providing early intervention for children from ages 0 to 6 years old. The goals also include developing a local multi-disciplinary diagnostic team capability and providing financial assistance for intervention services based on need. The development of this foundation involved careful assessment of community capacities, locating community members who were willing to support and volunteer for the organization, and ensuring that services would not duplicate those already available. A capabilities approach was used to examine what might be possible given existing resources and what potential "unfreedoms" (barriers) may present themselves. Community members were empowered to participate as they volunteered their time and skills, while improving the quality of life of those families living with an autistic child.

This organization grew from one person listening to the needs of the identified community (families living with autism) and their aspirations. After assessing community capacities, including resources and supports required, the organization blossomed into a strong, volunteer-based group that has a diverse board of directors, a development committee, and a parent resource and support group. They are currently in the process of developing a local multi-disciplinary assessment team to alleviate the lengthy waiting period currently experienced by many families. This example demonstrates that community leadership can begin simply and expand into a larger enterprise as community members recognize the merit of the program and contribute their skills and abilities.

Linking Community Leadership and the Future of Occupational Therapy

Fieldwork educators play a critical leadership role in nurturing future occupational therapy practitioners, researchers, and leaders during the level II fieldwork experience. Fieldwork educators introduce students to various occupational therapy clinical and client communities. They contribute to the community of occupational therapy professionals, the community of clients, and the occupational therapy profession. Throughout the fieldwork education process, these educators assess the capabilities of students and build on student capacities in order to address student needs. They also provide opportunities for students to integrate the academic concept of evidence-based practice into clinical practice.

The future of occupational therapy rests in the hands of today's fieldwork students. Patricia Crist reminded occupational therapy fieldwork educators at the Metropolitan Occupational Therapy Education Council Joint Clinical Conference that level II fieldwork students will enter their facilities with the skills to support clinical research efforts, thus supporting the broader occupational therapy community, and beginning their journey along the path toward leadership.[49] Community leadership theory can provide fieldwork educators with the skills and tools to approach program/hospital administrators to request support for research efforts within the clinical or community setting. Creating these links between research and evidence-based practice, occupational therapy fieldwork education and community leadership will empower both occupational therapists and the occupational therapy profession.

Groups such as the Metropolitan Occupational Therapy Education Council of New York and New Jersey (MOTEC) demonstrate leadership in fieldwork education by providing a forum to discuss fieldwork issues by supporting fieldwork educators to stay current with evolving AOTA and the Accreditation Council for Occupational Therapy Education (ACOTE) standards. In addition, initiatives such as the Voluntary Credentialing for Fieldwork Educators (VCFWE) proposal, which was approved by the Representative Assembly at the 2008 annual AOTA Conference in Long Beach, California,[5] should have a unifying effect on the occupational therapy profession. This initiative will include voluntary training, the trainer programs, and a voluntary fieldwork educator's credentialing process. This is an important leadership effort that has the potential to elevate the status of our fieldwork educators while supporting their efforts. It will also serve to create more unified standards in the fieldwork education process while closing existing gaps between the association and fieldwork educators and between academic and fieldwork education.

Interdisciplinary Collaboration

The founders of the occupational therapy profession were physicians, architects, social workers, secretaries, nurses, etc.[50] From their different perspectives, each observed the effects of occupation in his or her individual environments and believed in its healing powers.[27] As in the days of our founders, occupation is gaining interdisciplinary appeal at the international level.[51] With the dawning of OS, the value of occupation as a means toward health is becoming more widely recognized by other disciplines.[51] Occupational therapists now have the opportunity to assert their leadership as the original purveyors of the relationship between occupation and health. Organizations such as the NIH provide support for health initiatives that take place at the community level. In some instances, interdisciplinary groups are incorporating Sen's Capabilities Approach to PAR initiatives within the community. Interdisciplinary teams such as the Center to Study Recovery in Social Contexts will collaborate to implement community health programs funded by the NIH. Thus, it will become increasingly important for occupational therapists to submit proposals for health initiatives. It will also be important to join interdisciplinary teams in planning and implementing these community health efforts. Strengthened by their interdisciplinary foundations and a broader perspective, occupational therapists can apply Sen's Capabilities Approach to establish the relevance of occupational therapy in the areas of health, well-being, and prevention.

Cross Publications and Joint Publications

As occupational therapists begin to engage in the necessary research to promote the occupational therapy profession, cross publications will provide a means to convey to other disciplines the valuable service that occupational therapists provide. Collaborative interdisciplinary publications can also extend recognition of the occupational therapy profession. Community leadership skills can help occupational therapists recognize and forge the necessary and diverse venues for cross and joint publications to promote the benefits of occupational therapy to a broader readership. A prime example of this cross publication is the *Occupational Therapy for Independent Living Older Adults: A Randomized Controlled Trial*, which was published in *JAMA*.[24]

In this well elderly study, Clark et al demonstrated significant benefits for preventative occupation in mitigating health risks related to various health functions and quality of life domains.[24] This was a significant body of work in promoting the value of occupation-centered occupational therapy services. The cost effectiveness of the Lifestyle Redesign[25] approach was also demonstrated as a result of this study. This publication of an occupational therapy approach in a widely recognized medical journal providing the highest level of evidence for the efficacy of occupational therapy practice led to funding and world recognition of occupational therapy as a formidable entity in health care.

Recognizing the Right Time to Take the Lead

Community leadership occurs when individuals prepare to take the lead. Fidler addressed necessary changes in occupational therapy education for establishing occupational therapists in community practice.[14] She considered occupational therapy as a key component in community health, and believed that the "community is tailor-made for such learning and for demonstrating the efficacy of occupational therapy."[1] Fidler understood the opportunities that were open to occupational therapists within a community setting, and her life work was an illustration of her visionary leadership and active participation in a broader health arena.

As occupational therapists recognize opportunities to take the lead, they will maintain current practice environments and emerge as leaders in new environments. For example, as occupational therapists review and build upon the work of AJ Ayres, they maintain and expand the profession's expertise in diagnosis and treatment of sensory processing disorders and assume leadership roles in doing so.

Researchers and scholars in the area of sensory integration responded to calls for leadership. A dedicated and diverse group responded to challenges from other disciplines regarding use of the sensory integration approach in occupational therapy intervention. As criticism grew, they recognized that a unified and organized body of research would be necessary in order to defend this practice area. Many occupational therapy scholars and researchers took the lead and updated AJ Ayres' 1972 theory of sensory integration to include current research in neuroscience as well as clarifications in terminology and diagnostic categories.[52]

Other occupational therapy practice areas face similar challenges. Dr. Nadine Revheim, a research scientist and licensed psychologist for the Nathan S. Kline Institute for Psychiatric Research in Orangeburg, New York, spent the earlier part of her career as an occupational therapist in mental health and worked for over 20 years in that capacity in a variety of psychiatric inpatient and outpatient settings. In a conversation with Dr. Revheim about occupational therapy's loss of ground in the area of mental health, Dr. Revheim recounted her frustration in observing that leadership roles were not always assumed by occupational therapists despite the multiple opportunities that were presented in team meetings (Revheim, personal communication, March 5, 2008).

Will the profession reclaim lost contributions in mental health? Will occupational therapists forge new ground in community health? If occupational therapists provide a valuable health service due to our central focus on occupation, is it our ethical obligation to bring this service to the attention of those who may benefit? If so, then we need to gain leadership skills to lead this effort in multiple community environments.

Current Occupational Therapy Community Leadership and Centennial Vision Creating an Occupation-Centered Community Health Leadership Plan will enable occupational therapists to move forward in leadership within community settings. In developing your Occupation-Centered Community Health Leadership Plan, you may want to consider some of these elements from the AOTA's Centennial Vision[53]:

- *Expanded collaboration for success*: We envision that occupational therapy is a critical partner in expanded alliances concerned with health and wellness locally and globally.

- *The power to influence*: We envision that the occupational therapy profession will have the power to influence decisions and key decision makers to enhance the profession and the lives and participation of the people we serve.

- *Membership is a professional responsibility*: We envision that AOTA membership is an implicit professional responsibility of the occupational therapy community.

- *A well-prepared diverse workforce*: We envision that the occupational therapy profession will have a well-prepared diverse workforce to meet society's occupational needs.

- *A clear, compelling image*: We envision that the occupational therapy profession will be the provider of choice for challenges related to everyday life and occupations.

- *Customers demand occupational therapy*: We envision that society recognizes the contribution of occupational therapy to health and wellness and demands access to services.

- *Evidence-based decision making*: We envision that providers, payers, and consumers of occupational therapy utilize readily available evidence in decision making.

- *Science-fostered innovation in occupational therapy practice*: We envision that science will be successful in competitive, interdisciplinary arenas that give understanding to guide our practice.

The WHO's *Disability and Rehabilitation Action Plan, 2006-2011*[54] is also helpful in developing an occupation-oriented community plan. The mission is to enhance the quality of life for persons with disabilities through national, regional, and global efforts to:

- Raise awareness about the magnitude and consequences of disability

- Facilitate data collection and analyze or disseminate disability-related data and information

- Support, promote, and strengthen health and rehabilitation services for persons with disabilities and their families

- Promote community-based rehabilitation (CBR)

- Promote development, production, distribution, and servicing of assistive technology

- Support the development, implementation, measurment, and monitoring of policies to improve the rights and opportunities for people with disabilities

- Build capacity among health and rehabilitation policymakers and service providers

- Foster multisectoral networks and partnerships

Establishing an Understanding of Occupational Therapy in the Community

It is useful to consider the critical impact of defining occupational therapy in every day community practice. Language and identity are inextricably linked. Some linguists have argued that our thinking is determined by language.[55] In explaining occupational therapy to the public, the language must reflect the core or philosophical base of the profession. The profession's unique contribution to health is occupation. Occupational therapists serve the occupational needs of individuals and the community. Is your practice occupation-centered? Should therapists actively encourage questions about why we are called occupational therapists? How comfortable are you in answering this question? What is occupational therapy?

It is essential to clarify occupational therapy's unique contribution to health for the professional community and the community at large. As occupational therapists assume roles as community leaders, they will be empowered to clearly articulate the tenets of the profession to clients, the general public, health care workers, educators, administrators, insurance companies, media, and policymakers. The contribution of occupation to the health and well-being of a person can be more easily conveyed from a position of leadership, and the necessary evidence for this contribution can be more widely established.

Reflection Activity

1. Establish a strong foundation—reflect upon Table 4-2. Draw comparisons from other leadership theories (described elsewhere in this book) to the occupational therapy theory for practice that you feel most drawn to. For example, if the Model of Human Occupation (MOHO)[56] resonates most strongly with you, which leadership theory might best fit for your community plan?
   - What common qualities and constructs do they share?
   - Apply them to your community leadership plan (below).
2. Do I really have the potential to be a leader? Refer to Chapter 2, *Discovering the Leader in You*, by Jan G. Garbarini to assess your capacity for leadership.
3. Who are you within the context of your community? Who would you like to be? Explore your perceptions of who you are within the context of community. What roles do you carry out on a daily basis?
4. Using the following concepts, compare your current role within the community to your desired role. After you have answered these questions, try to think in terms of how your desired role could fit into Sen's Capabilities Approach[35]:
   - Occupational therapists as agents of change
   - Occupational therapists as facilitators of the empowerment process of marginalized groups
   - Occupational therapists as facilitators of capacity building and increased organizational capacity
5. Would you consider accepting the role of community occupational therapy consultant and assisting community leaders and members to engage in PAR based on a community-identified occupational need? Questions to consider in comparing your current role to assuming the role of a community leader are as follows:
   - Which of the roles are likely to have a greater long-term impact on the client?

- Which of the roles are likely to be sustained by diverse and multiple funding sources?
- Which of these roles are likely to support the understanding of occupational therapy's unique contribution to health: "occupation," as well as the growth and survival of the occupational therapy profession?

Learning Activities

Develop a community leadership plan, beginning with a vision statement. Consider the following practice settings as you develop your plan:

- Early intervention
- School-based practice
- Adult (community health clubs, development of foundations, mature adult, or possibly programming at an independent living center)

Within your plan, include a projected timeline of your personal and professional community leadership goals, and outline the steps required to get you there:

- *One year*: Develop your vision statement, identify community capacities and needs related to your vision, and develop small goal statements to achieve each month. For example, in developing a local nonprofit community foundation, first steps will include writing vision, mission, and goal statements; completing a 501c3 application to obtain nonprofit status; building an organizational structure beginning with a board of directors; and recruiting active volunteers.

- *Five years*: Consider expanding your vision statement to address future growth and re-evaluate mission and goals, identify additional supports within the community to enhance the health of your community plan and the steps to sustain it, and groom others to assume leadership roles. For example, as the organization builds strength, reassess the original mission and goal statements. Are they still aligned with community needs? In the case of the Lowcountry Autism Foundation, the founders listened to the community and learned that in addition to financial support, early identification, and intervention, families were also very interested in respite care and recreational opportunities for their autistic children.

- *Ten years*: Consider the strength of your legacy, re-evaluate mission and goals, and consider expanding and sharing leadership roles. Is the plan self-sustaining? Does it need modification?

References

1. Fidler GS. Community practice: it's more than geography. In: Velde BP, Wittman PP. *Community Occupational Therapy Education and Practice*. New York, NY: Routledge; 2001.
2. Hancock T. The evolution, impact, and significance of the Healthy Cities/Communities Movement. *J Public Health Policy*. 1993;14(1):5-18.
3. Goodspeed SW. *Community Stewardship: Applying the Five Principles of Contemporary Governance*. Chicago, IL: AHA Press; 1998.
4. American Occupational Therapy Association. Occupational therapy practice framework: domain and process. *Am J Occup Ther*. 2002;56:609-639.
5. American Occupational Therapy Association. Occupational therapy practice framework: domain and process. 2nd ed. *Am J Occup Ther*. 2008;62:625-683.
6. World Health Organization. *International Classification of Functioning, Disability and Health (ICF)*. Geneva, Switzerland: Author; 2001.
7. Labonte R. Community development and the forms of authentic partnerships. In: Minkler M, ed. *Community Organizing and Community Building for Health*. 2nd ed. New Brunswick, NJ: Rutgers University Press; 2005.
8. World Health Organization. *Constitution of the World Health Organization*. 45th ed. Geneva, Switzerland: Author; 2006.

9. Grady A. Building inclusive community: a challenge for occupational therapy, 1994 Eleanor Clarke Slagle Lecture. *Am J Occup Ther.* 1995;49(4):300-310.

10. Law M, Cooper B, Strong S, Stewart D, Rigby P, Letts L. The person-environment-occupation model: a transactive approach to occupational performance. *Can J Occup Ther.* 1996;63(1):9-23.

11. Baum C, Law M. Community health: a responsibility, an opportunity, and a fit for occupational therapy. *Am J Occup Ther.* 1998;52(1):7-10.

12. West W. 1967 Eleanor Clarke Slagle lecture. In: Padilla R, ed. Professional responsibility in times of change. *Am J Occup Ther.* 1968;22(1):9-15.

13. Fidler GS. Learning as a growth process: a conceptual framework for professional education, 1965 Eleanor Clarke Slagle Lecture. *Am J Occup Ther.* 1966;20:1-8.

14. Fidler GS. The issue is: beyond the therapy model: building our future. *Am J Occup Ther.* 2000;54:99-101.

15. Fidler G. Learning as a growth process: a conceptual framework for professional education. In: Padilla R, ed. *A Professional Legacy: The Eleanor Clarke Slagle Lectures in Occupational Therapy, 1955-2004.* Bethesda, MD: American Occupational Therapy Association, Inc; 2005;54(1):115-126.

16. Ludwig F. Gail Fidler. In: Walker K, Ludwig F, eds. *Perspectives on Theory for the Practice of Occupational Therapy.* 3rd ed. Austin, TX: Pro-Ed; 2004.

17. West W. 1967 Eleanor Clarke Slagle lecture: professional responsibility in times of change. In: Padilla R, ed. A Professional Legacy: The Eleanor Clarke Slagle Lectures in Occupational Therapy, 1955-2004, 2nd ed. *American Journal of Occupational Therapy.* 2005;XXII(1):141-151.

18. American Occupational Therapy Association. Federal news highlights. 2008. Available at: http://www.aota.org/Practitioners/Advocacy/Federal/Highlights.aspx. Accessed June 12, 2008.

19. SPD Foundation. Advocacy: DSM-V initiative. 2008. Available at: http://www.spdfoundation.net/dsmv.html. Accessed June 16, 2008.

20. Northouse P. *Leadership: Theory and Practice.* 4th ed. Thousand Oaks, CA: Sage Publications; 2007.

21. Burns JM. *Leadership.* New York, NY: Harper & Row; 1978.

22. Fazio LS. *Developing Occupation-Centered Programs for the Community.* 2nd ed. Upper Saddle River, NJ: Prentice Hall; 2008.

23. Zemke R, Clark F. Preface. In: Zemke R, Clark F, eds. *Occupational Science: The Evolving Discipline.* Philadelphia, PA: F.A. Davis; 1996:vii-xviii.

24. Clark F, Azen S, Zemke R, et al. Occupational therapy for independent living older adults: a randomized controlled trial. *JAMA.* 1997;278(16):1321-1326.

25. University of Southern California. Lifestyle Redesign. 2008. Available at: http://www.usc.edu/schools/ihp/ot/about/faculty_practice/lifestyle.html. Accessed May 22, 2008.

26. Mandel DR, Jackson JM, Zempke R, Nelson L, Clark FA. *Lifestyle Redesign: Implementing the Well Elderly Program.* Bethesda, MD: American Occupational Therapy Association Press; 1999.

27. Peloquin SM. Occupational therapy service: individual and collective understandings of the founders. *Am J Occup Ther.* 1991;45:352-360.

28. Law M, Baum C, Dunn W. *Measuring Occupational Performance: Supporting Best Practice in Occupational Therapy.* 2nd ed. Thorofare, NJ: SLACK Incorporated; 2005:374-384.

29. Schkade J, Schultz S. Occupational adaptation: toward a holistic approach to contemporary practice, part 1. *Am J Occup Ther.* 1992;46(9):829-837.

30. Schultz S, Schkade J. Occupational adaptation: toward a holistic approach for contemporary practice, part 2. *Am J Occup Ther.* 1992;46(10):917-925.

31. Murray JB, Klinger L, McKinnon C. The deaf: an exploration of their participation in community life. *OTJR: Occupation, Participation and Health.* 2007;27(3):113-120.

32. Hersey P, Blanchard K, Johnson DE. *Management of Organizational Behavior: Utilizing Human Resources.* 7th ed. Englewood Cliffs, NJ: Prentice-Hall; 1996.

33. Kouzes J, Posner B. *The Leadership Challenge.* 4th ed. San Francisco, CA: Jossey-Bass; 2007.

34. Schkade J, Schultz S. Occupational adaptation. In: Kramer P, Hinjosa J, Royeen CB, eds. *Perspectives in Human Occupation: Participation in Life.* Philadelphia, PA: Lippincott Williams & Wilkins; 2003.

35. Sen A. *Development as Freedom.* New York, NY: Random House; 1999.

36. Hopper K. Rethinking social recovery in schizophrenia: what a capabilities approach might offer. *Soc Sci Med.* 2007;65:868-879.

37. Moyers P. *Presidential Address.* Paper presented at the American Occupational Therapy Association Annual Conference, Long Beach, CA; April 11, 2008.

38. Whiteford G. Occupational deprivation: global challenge in the new millennium. *Br J Occup Ther.* 2000;63(5):200-204.

39. Mitra S. *The Capabilities Approach: An Introduction.* Paper presented at the Capabilities Seminar, Center for Urban and Community Services, East Harlem, NY; November 28, 2008.

40. Lipowski Z. Delirium, clouding of consciousness and confusion. *J Nerv Ment Dis.* 1967;145(2):245.

41. Neufield P, Kniepmann K. Gateway to wellness: an occupational therapy collaboration with the National Multiple Sclerosis Society. In: Velde BP, Wittman PP. *Community Occupational Therapy Education and Practice.* New York, NY: Routledge; 2001.

42. Minkler M, Wallerstein N. Improving health through community organization and community building: a health education perspective. In: Minkler M. *Community Organizing and Community Building for Health.* 2nd ed. New Brunswick, NJ: Rutgers University Press; 2005:26-50.

43. Robbins SP, Chatterjee P, Canda ER. *Contemporary Human Behavior Theory.* Boston, MA: Allyn & Bacon; 1998.

44. Arai S. Empowerment: from the theoretical to the personal. *J Leisurability*. 1997;24(1):1-9.
45. Balcazar FE, Keys CB, Kaplan DL, Suarez-Balcazar Y. Participatory action research and people with disabilities: principles and challenges. *Can J Rehabil*. 1998;12(2):105-112.
46. Letts L. Occupational therapy and participatory research: a partnership worth pursuing. *Am J Occup Ther*. 2003;57(1):77-87.
47. Taylor R, Braveman B, Hammel J. Developing and evaluating community based services through participatory action research: two case examples. *Am J Occup Ther*. 2004;58(1):73-82.
48. Suarez-Balcazar Y. Empowerment and participatory evaluation of a community health intervention: implications for occupational therapy. *OTJR: Occupation, Participation and Health*. 2005;25(4):133-142.
49. Crist Patricia. *Presentation*. Presented at the Annual Joint Clinical Council Day of the Metropolitan Occupational Therapy Education Council (MOTEC) of NY and NJ. New York University, New York, NY; December 5, 2007.
50. Johnson J. Old values-new directions: competence, adaptation, integration. *Am J Occup Ther*. 1981;35(9):589-598.
51. Wood W. Nationally speaking: it is jump time for occupational therapy. *Am J Occup Ther*. 1998;52(6):403-411.
52. Miller LJ, Anzalone M, Lane S, Cermak S, Osten E. Concept evolution in sensory integration: a proposed nosology for diagnosis. *Am J Occup Ther*. 2007;61(2):135-140.
53. American Occupational Therapy Association. AOTA's centennial vision and executive summary. *Am J Occup Ther*. 2006;61(6):613-614.
54. World Health Organization. Disability and rehabilitation action plan, 2006-2011. 2006. Available at: http://www.who.int/disabilities/en/. Accessed May 22, 2007.
55. Bowers CA. *The Cultural Dimensions of Educational Computing: Understanding the Non-Neutrality of Technology*. New York, NY: Teachers College Press; 1988.
56. Kielhofner G. *A Model of Human Occupation: Theory and Application*. Philadelphia, PA: Lippincott Williams & Wilkins; 2008.

Suggested Readings

American Occupational Therapy Association. Occupational therapy practice framework: domain and process. *Am J Occup Ther.* 2008;56(6):609-639.

Balcazar FE, Keys CB, Suarez-Balcazar Y. Empowering Latinos with disabilities to address issues of independent living and disability rights: a capacity-building approach. *J Prev Interv Community.* 2001;21(2):53-70.

Baum MC. Presidential Address, 2006: centennial challenges, millennium opportunities. *Am J Occup Ther.* 2006;60(6):609-616.

Bowers CA. *The Cultural Dimensions of Educational Computing: Understanding the Non-Neutrality of Technology.* New York, NY: Teachers College Press; 1998.

Cockburn L, Trentham B. Participatory action research: integrating community occupational therapy practice and research. *Can J Occup Ther.* 2002;69(1):20-30.

Fazio LS. *Developing Occupation-Centered Programs for the Community: A Workbook for Students and Professionals.* Upper Saddle River, NJ: Prentice Hall; 2000.

Gilkeson GE. *Occupational Therapy Leadership: Marketing Yourself, Your Profession, and Your Organization.* Philadelphia, PA: F.A. Davis Company; 1997.

Hooper K, Thomas Y, Clarke M. Health professional partnerships and their impact on aboriginal health: an occupational therapist's and aboriginal health worker's perspective. *Aust J Rural Health.* 2007;15:46-51.

Howard BS. How high do we jump? The effect of reimbursement on occupational therapy. *Am J Occup Ther.* 1991;45(10):875-881.

Johnson J. Old values-new directions: competence, adaptation, integration. *Am J Occup Ther.* 1981;35(9):589-598.

Larson E, Wood W, Clark F. Occupational science: building the science and practice of occupation through an academic discipline. In: Crepeau EB, Cohn ES, Boyt Schell BA. *Willard & Spackman's Occupational Therapy.* 10th ed. Philadelphia, PA: Lippincott Williams & Wilkins; 2003:15-26.

Minkler M. *Community Organizing and Community Building for Health.* 2nd ed. New Brunswick, NJ: Rutgers University Press; 2005.

Velde BP, Wittman PP. *Community Occupational Therapy Education and Practice.* New York, NY: Routledge; 2002.

Ware NC, Hopper D, Tugenberg T, Dickey B, Fisher D. Connectedness and citizenship: redefining social integration. *Psychiatr Serv.* 2007;58(4):469-574.

West W. 1980 Eleanor Clarke Slagle lecture: a reaffirmed philosophy and practice of occupational therapy for the 1980s. *Am J Occup Ther.* 1984;38(1):15-23.

Whiteford G. Occupational deprivation: global challenge in the new millennium. *Br J Occup Ther.* 2000;63(5):200-204.

Wood W. The issue is: it is jump time for occupational therapy. *Am J Occup Ther.* 1998;52(6):403-406.

Leadership in the Occupational Therapy Classroom

Teresa Plummer, MSOT, OTR, ATP

Learning Objectives

1. Describe the responsibilities of the occupational therapy educator and occupational therapy student.
2. Identify specific leadership theories that can be applied to academic settings.
3. Describe guidelines for desired participation in the classroom setting.

> *Don't tell people how to do things, tell them what to do*
> *and let them surprise you with the results.*
> —George S. Patton

Occupational therapists practice in a complex health care environment. Preparing students to enter this arena requires a thorough understanding of the demands and expectations of the health care system, the human service system, and the personal and professional skills necessary to interact effectively with others. Further, it requires that occupational therapists demonstrate leadership and collaboration with clients, families, and other health care providers. Leadership is a collaborative process designed to achieve a specific goal.[1] In an academic environment, the specific goal is to educate the future occupational therapist. Leadership skills are a prerequisite for the occupational therapy educator.

Educators need to understand competency standards. This includes the definitions and the processes of a student's acquisition of competencies and the non-cognitive and cognitive components of competencies. The rapidly changing and dynamic health care service delivery systems require occupational therapy students to develop skills and knowledge for clinical practice, advocacy, education, management, research, and leadership.[2] For the occupational therapy profession, this involves imparting cognitive skills and knowledge as well as professional socialization, empathy, and leadership. Occupational therapy educators may find it helpful to have an understanding of leadership theories, skills, and strategies.

This chapter will discuss several leadership theories that have implications for the classroom. Additionally, this chapter will discuss the responsibility of educators to effectively demonstrate and teach leadership in the classroom by means of modeling, mentorship, and practice. Finally, this chapter will discuss specific approaches to developing an atmosphere of leadership, communication, and motivation.

The Occupational Therapy Student

The developmental tasks associated with early adulthood include the following[3]:

- Achieve independence from his or her family of origin.
- Develop identity on the basis of self-worth.
- Develop the ability to share one's inner self with others.
- Find something higher than self to believe in.
- Develop satisfying social relationships.
- Balance expression of personal needs and interests with cultural expectations.
- Assume responsibility for independent decision making.
- Develop expertise in chosen career

Changes that occur at this age persist into adulthood and thereby may influence one's actions and career choices.[4] For the occupational therapy student, these dimensions contribute to the development of interpersonal skills. Milton discusses the role of mentorship in an effort to impart leadership skills.[5] "Mentorship is a multidimensional concept of coming to know through purposeful processes of leading-following, which has connotations of teacher, overseer, coach, and one who provides support."[5] To interact in a mentorship relationship is to coparticipate in an unfolding drama or art of leadership. The process of mentorship, a role consistent with educator-student, is to help students prioritize and live their values and beliefs moment to moment, while uniquely upholding personal integrity.[5] It is through this process that the core values of occupational therapy are hand delivered to a new generation of occupational therapists.

Occupational therapy students are adult learners. Knowles et al noted that scholars of adult learning theories indicate few basic assumptions regarding adult learners.[6] A review of these 6 assumptions may be helpful in discussing leadership in the academic environment. Adult learners need to know why they should learn the subject at hand.[6] This requires that the educator articulate the rationale for why the student must know the material and how it will benefit the student. It may be helpful for the student to reflect on his or her learning needs, goals, and role in the learning process. This suggests that students are active learners, contributing to the goals and objectives of the material and reflecting upon their successful attainment of the knowledge and skill.

Knowles et al emphasize that adult learners desire to be autonomous, yet may be dependent learners based on their prior educational experience.[6] It is helpful for the educator to distinguish between a student's self-motivation and self-directed learning. While a student may be very motivated to learn and apply the material, he or she may not have the skills to determine the path of inquiry for self-directed learning. The educator may need to adjust his or her level of direction and support based on the student's ability to be self-directed in his or her learning.

Adult learners use their experiences to learn new material.[6] For the occupational therapy student, most of the experience is educational rather than clinical. Students may find it helpful and motivating to hear clinical examples from the perspective of the educator to bring life into occupational therapy education. This provides the educator an opportunity to share his or her clinical experiences and reveal the heart of occupational therapy. By illustrating clinical examples, an educator provides students with a vision of the end result of their learning.

Adult learners are more apt to be motivated to learn new material when they need to know the subject matter. Occupational therapy students engaged in concurrent clinical fieldwork or utilizing case studies as assigned work may be more prone to ask questions and be self-directed and motivated to learn when the need to apply the information is concurrent with the teaching of new material. Learning is a hierarchical process of new knowledge building upon previous knowledge. It may be beneficial to the student to recognize this as they apply both previously covered materials with new material. For instance, the student may have learned the spinal tracts in a neurology course and apply the pathophysiology of this topic in a rehabilitation intervention course. This particular example illustrates the overlapping nature of occupational therapy education.

Adults are task- or problem-centered in their learning orientation.[6] Learning may be more effective if students understand how the skill or knowledge can be used to answer a question or solve a problem. It may be helpful if students reflect on their learning needs in relation to a task to be accomplished or a skill to be mastered.

A final assumption regarding adult learners reflects on the students' motivation to learn. Knowles et al suggest that adult learners are intrinsically motivated, though they may also be motivated by external factors.[6] That is to say, while the occupational therapy student is motivated to demonstrate his or her knowledge by reflecting upon his or her grade, he or she is more motivated to learn material that can be applied to clinical practice areas of interest.

Kang offers a postmodern view of adult learning by creating a way for educators to understand the complexity of learning outside of traditional learning theories.[7] Through the use of activity observation that can occur anytime and anywhere, the adult learner has opportunities to make connections between information gained and real life experiences. Multiple and varied ways of approaching situations is supported and even expected within this framework of adult learning.[7]

The occupational therapy educator and student are encouraged to fully understand learning theories and models, though this is not within the scope of this chapter. It is, however, helpful to reflect upon learning theories and the implications these may have upon leadership in the academic setting. The reader will be encouraged to explore this topic at the conclusion of this chapter.

Leadership in the Academic Environment

Leadership is a highly valued, complex phenomenon that is difficult to conceptualize.[1] The leadership process requires leaders and followers who act in accordance within their established values, attitudes, and skills. While leadership occurs within a specific context, it can and usually is a trait, skill, or practice that has adaptability over a range of contexts. Typically, in the academic environment, the instructor is the leader and the students are the followers. It may be suggested that this is not always the case or the desired outcome. In an effort to impart professional skills and behaviors, it may be helpful for the instructor to model or demonstrate leadership skills. In other words, this deliberate process should be undertaken by the instructor with respect for the formative potential and lasting impression that this instills on the student. Therefore, it may be helpful to review a few of the well-known leadership theories.

Leadership Theory

Transformational Leadership

Transformational leadership is particularly relevant in occupational therapy education because it is a process that transforms or changes individuals. This is particularly significant for young adults who are in a rapid state of transformation by virtue of age as previously discussed.

Transformational leadership is concerned with emotions, values, ethics, goals, and motivation.[1] The leader plays a significant role in precipitating change, though the leader and follower are allies with an expressed mission to accomplish. In an educational context, transformational leadership seeks to motivate students to achieve more than is expected by raising consciousness about the value of learning. It aims to encourage the student to transcend his or her self-interest in view of developing his or her professional identity.[1] This is particularly applicable in occupational therapy education where a student is typically within a specified cohort of others during the entire professional education.

Developing professional identity occurs over time and within various contexts. For this reason, students may exhibit leadership attributes in one particular class but not another. Developing professional socialization and leadership begins when the student enters the academic environment and intensifies as the student begins to make the transition from classroom to practice setting.[8] Students may emulate the educator to "try out" their newly acquired professional identity. Educators have great opportunity to shape the student and the profession by respectfully providing feedback concerning professional socialization skills and leadership attributes to the student. Likewise, students are encouraged to establish their professional identity as they move from a role of student to clinician. The academic environment should be a safe and nurturing arena for such development.

Team Leadership

Teams are organizational groups consisting of interdependent individuals that have a common goal.[1] It is through collaborative efforts rather than the collective efforts of each individual that the goals are realized. In the classroom, this theory can be applied through experiential learning tasks such as problem-based case studies or practice skills such as splinting. The instructor/leader can assume a less visible role while the students develop strategies for addressing a specific task. Zaccaro et al propose that leadership is the essential driver and influences the team through 4 processes[9]:

1. Cognitive
2. Motivational
3. Effective
4. Coordination

The instructor helps the students cognitively understand the problem, providing adequate theoretical and foundational knowledge related to the activity. The motivational component helps the team to stay organized, congruent, and cohesive by setting achievable yet high performance standards. The instructor may work as a member of the team to provide adequate supervision and skill acquisition. The effective role of the instructor is to provide clear goals, strategies, skills, and specified behavioral and action strategies to achieve the ultimate goals. Additionally, the instructor/leader coordinates the activity by matching the member's skills with the activity, providing feedback and direction and modifying the task or the environment for successful task achievement. Finally, the role of the leader is to maintain focus, create a collaborative climate, build confidence among the team, demonstrate competency in the activity, and manage and direct the ultimate group performance.

Case Example

Occupational Therapy Students

Occupational therapy students in their third semester are assigned a group task in their "Assistive Technology III—Pediatric Practice" course. The goal is to build a scaled model of an accessible playground. They are asked to nominate 3 members for the "planning commission," whose role is to assign tasks to all group members, schedule all meetings, and allocate monies of a prescribed budget.

- As a member of the occupational therapy class, what attributes, characteristics, and skills would you consider to be important for the members of the "planning commission?"
- Other members are responsible for determining the guidelines for accessibility, the materials needed, the design of the playground, or the literature review that supports the need for accessible playgrounds. What role would you be most suited for? What skills do you possess that would be helpful in fulfilling this role?
- Which tasks would be the most challenging for you? Describe ways that you can develop your skills in this area.

Occupational Therapy Educator

What role can you as an educator take in facilitating leadership skills among the commission and other team members?

Path-Goal Theory

Path-goal theory reflects on the role of the leader to motivate the followers to accomplish specified goals. The assertions of this theory include the leader's responsibility in defining the goals, clarifying the path, removing any obstacles, and providing necessary support.[10] Philosophically, the path-goal theory suggests that the leader find a style that best suits the needs of the followers and consider the goal and its inherent characteristics as being either structured or unstructured. This is similar to matching teaching and learning styles utilized in much of the didactic pedagogy. While path-goal theory is certainly an applicable theory for academic settings, it suggests that the follower is less active than other theoretical approaches such as team leadership.

Case Example

Occupational therapy students are required to demonstrate their competency in fabricating a static resting hand splint.

- Using the path-goal theory, what are the roles and responsibilities of the educator to direct the student?
- Provide examples of how the educator can motivate the student to accomplish this task.

Leader-Member Exchange Theory

The previous theories highlight leadership from the perspective of the leader, the follower, and the context. Leader-member exchange, as the name implies, conceptualizes leadership as an interaction between the leader and follower.[1] This theory emphasizes mutual trust, respect, and commitment between the leader and the subordinate. While this has potential for the post-professional level of education, the student and the instructor are professional peers. It may have limitations for some academic environments where the desired outcome is to encourage respect of authority. The instructor/leader may consider it necessary to establish communication guidelines that demonstrate a hierarchal level of communication.

Case Example

Small groups of occupational therapy students enrolled in "Critical Reasoning and Evidence-Based Practice" complete a poster for a classroom presentation. Several groups of students express an interest in presenting their posters at the state occupational therapy annual conference. The students approach the educator to assist them in fulfilling their interest.

- As one of these students, how would you describe the role of the educator in this situation?
- What characteristics of the educator would you find helpful?
- As an occupational therapy student, what is your responsibility in this relationship?
- Create an outline of responsibilities that conceptualize the role of the student and the educator and determine ways that these objectives can be measured.

Responsibility of Occupational Therapy Educators

Occupational therapy education aims to impart knowledge and skill while developing professional behaviors such as communication and leadership. Because most occupational therapy students are young adults, the attitudes, interest, values, professional skills, and character development that undergird clinical and professional behaviors is not fully developed.[11] This provides an opportunity for educators to be influential in the positive development of professional behaviors. Interpersonal and communication skills are in the effective domain of learning and are subjective in nature, making it difficult to quantify, yet they are considered critical for successful interaction with clients.[11-14]

While interpersonal skills are viewed as behavioral characteristics and actions, they are couched in the concept of "professional competency." Therefore, it is necessary to understand the theme of competency and competence as it relates to the characteristics of a profession. "Competencies are not a set of personal attributes, but rather encompass set of skills, knowledge, and abilities that collectively reflect the demands and goals of the organization or profession."[14]

The concept of professional competence has evolved over time from the one dimensional concept of knowledge or cognitive skills to a more multidimensional one involving knowledge and skills. More recently, educational research has empirically identified a third dimension of competency—interpersonal flexibility, or the ability to tolerate ambiguity and adapt interpersonal skills while intuitively sensing the need to do so. Such a definition broadens the concept of competency to include interpersonal skills and leadership. In other words, it is not just possessing the knowledge, but applying the knowledge under a variety of circumstances that require the practitioner to intuitively understand the environment, the audience, and the outcome of the interaction. Professional competence is complex and incorporates both formal and informal knowledge and the ability to make informed professional judgments.[15] Undeniably, an occupational therapist or occupational therapy student must possess a wide range of discipline-specific knowledge. Additionally, he or she must possess the interpersonal flexibility to apply such knowledge within a variety of practice arenas. There is a professional mandate that learning interpersonal and leadership skills is critical in the process of developing competencies for entry-level practice.[2]

While cognitive skills, competencies, and knowledge are relevant and important characteristics of the occupational therapy student and practitioner, emotional skills, professional behaviors, and leadership skills are required (particularly in clinical practice) in order for the occupational therapist to interact effectively with those to whom he or she provides care. Understanding the role of interpersonal skills and leadership may contribute to an enhanced appreciation toward the educational influence of occupational therapy students, particularly as it relates to clinical practice.

Leaders Motivate Performance and Values

Gouveia, commenting on the role of a pharmacy manager, suggests that excellence in practice depends in part on factors such as motivation to progress to higher levels, empowerment of all team members, and continuous innovation.[16] He indicates the need for interdisciplinary collaboration to articulate and practice pharmacy, guided by a moral compass that includes common values and a common vision with the goal of serving the client with wisdom. Such an ambition requires other health care practitioners to develop a professional culture that nurtures human interaction in an effort to develop interconnectedness and a thoughtful, team-centered creative vision.

Passion for Lifelong Learning

As occupational therapists, we are capable and responsible for developing our competency in clinical practice, leadership, and communication skills. Therefore, we are accountable for educating students to perform similarly. Health care organizations are in need of self-directed, personal, growth-oriented lifelong learners.[17] Professional development is a dynamic process for the clinician and student alike. It involves the acquisition of theoretical concepts and ideas, the application of values, and behaviors associated with professionalism. AOTA asserts, "Ensuring competence is the responsibility of everyone, including the individual practitioner, employers, professional associations, and regulatory boards. The key, however, rests with the individual who must be self-directed to attain and maintain competency."[18]

Developing self-initiated lifelong learning objectives is critical in order for an occupational therapist to maintain current professional development. Self-awareness and self-regulation are important components of an individual's ability to analyze their practice and commit to lifelong learning. The instructor/leader should possess, express, and model a lifelong learning commitment. In an academic setting, it may be the instructor or professor whose leadership skills may be emulated and therefore may perpetuate either negative or positive leadership traits.

Christie et al examined the influence of faculty on occupational therapy student's choice of specific practice area choice.[19] Using a random sample survey, they reviewed the findings of 131 recent occupational therapy graduates. They concluded that the instructor's interpersonal and attitudinal qualities have a great impact on the student. The instructor who had a positive influence was one that had clinical experience, was well-prepared, stimulated discussions, and was enthusiastic and provided feedback. This individual was viewed as a positive role model, exemplifying a supportive and encouraging demeanor toward students. This is compared to the instructor who had little clinical experience and was uncertain of theory, inconsistent, demonstrated little enthusiasm, non-supportive, and burned out.

Leaders Facilitate Rather Than Instruct

Haider, in discussing the role of a nurse as an educator, describes the teacher as a change agent.[20] The teacher's role is to facilitate rather than instruct, so education is about the transformation of the learner as a participant of his or her own education. Education is not a transfer of information, but a transformation of an individual. Such a concept defines leadership for both the student and the teacher. In this way, the instructor empowers the learner to take responsibility for active learning. Empowerment stimulates learning and growth of the individual.[21] An effective leader promotes personal growth to strengthen the learner's ability to tackle new tasks, learn new skills, and develop a sense of ownership for the learning process. This idea suggests that the leader have a commitment to the needs of the learner and measure his or her own achievement by measuring the developing skills of the learner.

Human Connectedness

While applied to leadership in clinical practice, appreciative inquiry is described by Moody et al as a model to facilitate renewal in the nursing profession.[22] The concepts are equally relevant in the field of occupational therapy and are worthy of consideration for the educator. They suggest that renewal involve an appreciation of the values that support interconnectedness and interrelationships. Such concepts are inherent in the philosophical assumptions of occupational therapy, which consider the holistic and positive view of human beings. Appreciative inquiry is a values-centered leadership style that encourages members of differing backgrounds, cultures, and viewpoints to focus on what works well rather than what is not working.[22] This particular relevant leadership style can be modeled, taught, and practiced in occupational therapy education arenas. Occupational therapy practitioners, in an effort to embrace a client-centered practice, may demonstrate skills that value diversity and highlight the strengths of the client, much like the appreciative inquiry model of leadership.

Experts in management recognize that one consistent and requisite feature that fosters the health of a complex organization is the appreciation of common values, which supports the interconnectedness of members of an organization.[22] Appreciative inquiry creates a language of understanding and interaction that celebrates diversity and creates a culture in which values are expressed, heard, and honored. The language of appreciation does not label a person, but rather recognizes the actions and exchanges that are enriching to an organization. Modeling this language in the classroom recognizes the efforts of the student and celebrates his or her contributions to a discussion. This attitude of acceptance allows others to express their viewpoint without fear of rebuttal or embarrassment. Ultimately, this may develop a student's capacity to respect, honor, and appreciate an opposing set of values and beliefs held by other practitioners or clients. Such leadership seeks to acknowledge the contributions of all members of a collective society without prejudice.

Establishing Leadership

Build a Leadership of Kindness

McIvor considers kindness a proactive approach in enhancing and sustaining the health of people within an organization.[17] This approach requires an influential leader to create a culture of kindness. She suggests that kindness is tripartite, involving kindness to oneself, kindness to colleagues, and kindness to the community. As occupational therapy educators modeling and teaching leadership, it is worthwhile to consider how these traits potentially contribute to developing a positive learning environment for students. Kindness is only a true trait if it arises from a genuine spirit of caring. It requires authenticity. An authentic person is aware of his or her own behaviors and knows his or her values and beliefs. Authenticity means you are genuine and not embarrassed to show humanness. Kindness to self includes traits such as authenticity, attitude, resilience, and excellence.[17] The academic culture has an opportunity to nurture and support such attributes in students in order to enhance their potential to become effective leaders.

Further, educators should seek opportunities to facilitate students to demonstrate kindness to colleagues such as trust, compassion, courage, and friendship.[17] This creates a climate conducive to learning and supporting one another and develops long-lasting relationships among students. Finally, kindness in the community involves traits such as service, responsibility, integrity, and tolerance.[17] Collectively, these traits are characteristic of leadership attributes that should be cultivated and taught as part of the professional preparation of occupational therapists.

Emotional Intelligence

Emotional intelligence consists of 4 fundamental skills: self-awareness, self-management, social awareness, and social skills.[23] Emotional intelligence is a core concept related to one's ability to reason with one's emotions in relation to self and others.[24] A therapist-client interaction is affected by emotional intelligence. Every human contact may result in a positive or negative experience. In the moment, it can be healing or harmful. Occupational therapy education should focus on the value and development of emotions as a core construct of a therapeutic relationship with client-therapist, instructor-student. When teachers fail to pay attention to emotional development, they neglect the significance of human relationships.[24] Communication is an occupational therapy intervention similar to self-care or home management instruction. It is not enough to simply instruct students to develop practice interventions skills; we must teach communication skills. Freshwater and Stickley, referring to nursing education, contend that by separating communication training from the emotional context of human interaction, the art of nursing is reduced to the science of a technician.[24] This is equally applicable in the art of occupational therapy. Effective education that imbues emotional intelligence can contribute to effective learning, stimulate self-awareness and personal growth, and therefore transform the life and practice of occupational therapy and the student.

Health care professionals clearly interact with human emotion, whether it be through pain, celebration, discomfort, disappointment, sadness, grief, joy, or elation.[24] The ability to manage our own emotional life, interpret other people's emotions, and respond appropriately is a prerequisite for any health care provider. It is necessary for the leader/teacher to be willing, capable, and competent to explore the realm of emotional intelligence in an effort to teach students to explore and give voice to clients in regard to emotions. In order to do so, the teacher/leader should be in intimate contact with his or her own emotions and able to facilitate student learning from a position of self-reflection and self-knowledge. Finally, emotions and expressive modalities instantly penetrate the heart of learning. More critically, they distinguish the concepts of care and caring from the constructs of treatment and care.[24] Care and caring are the empathetic and understanding acts that occur in the context of human interconnectedness. The art of communication requires emotional intelligence.

Teamwork and Responsibility

The definition of a leader has changed in recent years in response to shifting health care practices.[25] The new paradigm of leadership recognizes that organizations are the sum of their interrelated parts and that the leader functions as mentor, coach, and leader. To prosper and flourish in this new paradigm, a leader should promote teamwork, shared governance, and mentorship.[25] The academic environment is certainly capable of supporting and teaching within this new leadership paradigm. In fact, occupational therapy educators have many opportunities to structure learning tasks that require students to practice shared governance through group projects. Instructors, by mentoring student projects, model the skills of coaching and mentorship that students will one day utilize in occupational therapy settings.

Case Example

Students enrolled in an "Introduction to Assistive Technology" course are assigned the task of measuring accessibility of the campus and its surrounding environs. The instructor/leader demonstrates this through a review of the accessibility guidelines found in the text. Further, the instructor highlights the legislative policies that have supported accessibility. Finally, the instructor demonstrates how the environment can be modified with technological applications. The students divide into groups of 3 and complete an accessibility checklist according to the Americans with Disabilities Act (ADA) compliance for public buildings of the entire campus and its related buildings. The students are expected to determine who will cover which buildings, when the project will be completed, and how the findings will be presented. In this example, the leader simply modeled one small aspect of the assignment and requested the students to determine how to apply this task to their assignment. What characteristics of the educator would you find helpful?

Guidelines for Participation

Shared Responsibility

Effective leadership highly regards the people of the organization; encourages shared responsibility; and expects high levels of participation, involvement, and commitment.[16] Expecting a high level of performance from students communicates the instructor's trust in the students' ability to perform. Granted, the level of expectation must parallel the student's potential to insure relative success. The converse, expecting less than students are capable of, communicates a lack of trust and may be demotivating to students. By expecting optimal commitment and participation from students, educators prepare the student for a professional level practice that is consistent with current health care needs. Educators impart professional values of teamwork, commitment, and diligence by setting the standard for classroom participation. Anything less than exceptional expectations devalues the potential contribution that a future practitioner will make upon the profession. Leadership in the classroom demonstrates, articulates, and values high levels of commitment and participation.

Keys for the Classroom

To model and instruct traits, it may be beneficial to provide a set of behavioral guidelines for students. This may be a helpful organizational tool for the occupational therapy educator. May and Norbury provide several guidelines for leadership training objectives, some of which may be applicable in a classroom setting.[26] Several suggested behavior guidelines are as follows.

Participants will[26]:
- Engage in honest and open communication.
- Develop effective relationships that will enable them to function effectively as part of multidisciplinary or multiprofessional teams.
- Recognize personal behaviors and the impact of these on others.
- Create visions and lead others toward them.
- Create cultures in which personal and departmental risktaking is encouraged.
- Become self-aware and evaluate personal performance through reflection and feedback.
- Provide feedback to others to ensure their development.
- Develop formal and informal networks in order to share views, experiences, and areas of good practice.

Developing a clear, measurable set of behavior guidelines allows the teacher and student to understand the desired actions. It allows for goal setting and acts as a means to determine success for behaviors. It may be helpful for the educator and student to collectively establish such guidelines at the beginning of a semester and re-evaluate the guidelines for necessary adjustments or changes for upcoming semesters.

Handling Mistakes

Failure is an inevitable part of life and provides a tremendous opportunity for growth[27] if handled with finesse and openness. For students, failures may come in the form of a less-than-perfect grade on an exam to a significant inability to master a particular skill. Regardless of the intensity, failures occur. Kerfoot states that a leader's ability to handle failure displays one's true character.[27] The occupational therapy student may have repeated opportunities to learn this skill.

It may be helpful for occupational therapy educators to monitor the development of a student's ability to grow through experiencing failures. Kerfoot states that leaders miss an opportunity to demonstrate courage, integrity, and values clarification when they fail to admit and deal with their failures.[27] I suggest the same is true for a student. Occupational therapy educators may provide an opportunity for students to discuss their personal perspectives on their failures. Students will make mistakes, as all people do. The uniqueness of the teacher-student relationship allows deliberate and insightful dialogue to take place. In this mentorship process, a student learns valuable leadership skills. Teaching a student rigorous accountability for actions and artful acceptance of failures is the art of an educator.

Summary

This chapter discusses the responsibility of the occupational therapy educator to model and teach leadership skills and strategies as core competencies for an entry-level occupational therapist. Because students are highly influenced, it is imperative that modeling, instruction, and feedback concerning leadership be an integral part of occupational therapy education.

Several leadership theories that apply to occupational therapy academic environment were presented. The transformational leadership theory is particularly relevant because it deals with emotions, values, ethics, and goals, which are all aspects of professional development in the occupational therapy student. Team leadership was highlighted because many occupational therapy practitioners function as members of an interdisciplinary team, reinforcing the need to teach in a team-oriented environment. The need for occupational therapists to demonstrate leadership puts the onus on the occupational therapy educator to model, instruct, and provide feedback in the development of occupational therapy in academic education.

Reflection Activity

After reading this chapter, you may have thoughts about how to demonstrate leadership in the classroom. Perhaps your future includes teaching in an occupational therapy curriculum. Take a few minutes and review the section on "Keys for the Classroom." Using this and other concepts covered in this chapter, write your "Creed for Teaching as a Leader." Your creed should represent your philosophy, your beliefs, and ultimately your commitment to teach as a leader. Your sentences within your creed should begin with phrases such as, "I believe..." You may share these among your peers and discuss ways that you may demonstrate your creed as a student learner, practicing occupational therapist, or academic educator.

Reflection Activity

1. This chapter reflected upon 6 assumptions of adult learning theories as presented by Knowles et al.[6] How are these learning assumptions similar or different from leadership theories?

2. Find 2 to 3 recent literature sources on adult learning and compare/contrast these to the Knowles et al assumptions.[6]

3. Identify 4 or 5 responsibilities of the "educator" and 4 or 5 responsibilities of the "student." Compare and contrast these characteristics.

4. Imagine that you are an occupational therapy educator developing a syllabus for your class. Within the syllabus, you list a set of desired behaviors for students. Referring to the "Keys for the Classroom" on page 76, what specific behaviors will you encourage?

5. Select one leadership theory discussed in this chapter. Identify the goals of this leadership theory as applied in the academic setting. Determine how these goals/objectives can be measured.

References

1. Northouse P. *Leadership: Theory and Practice*. Thousand Oaks, CA: Sage Publications; 2007.
2. American Occupational Therapy Association. Accreditation Council for Occupational Therapy Education (ACOTE) standards and interpretive guidelines. 2007. Available at: http:www.aota.org/Educate/Accredit/StandardsReview. Accessed May 15, 2007.
3. Schuster C, Ashburn S. *The Process of Human Development: A Holistic Life-Span Approach*. Philadelphia, PA: Lippincott Williams & Wilkins; 1992.
4. Plummer T. *An Evaluation of Attitudes Toward Individuals With Disabilities and Professional Behaviors*. Unpublished thesis. Nashville, TN: Belmont University; 2005.
5. Milton C. A graduate curriculum guided by human becoming: journeying with the possible. *Nurs Sci Q*. 2004;16:214-288.
6. Knowles M, Elmwood H, Swanson R. *The Modern Practice of Adult Education: From Andragogy to Pedagogy*. Englewood Cliffs, NJ: Cambridge Adult Education; 1998.
7. Kang DJ. Rhizoactivity: toward a postmodern theory of lifelong learning. *Adult Educ Q*. 2007;57:205-220.
8. Koenig K. *Academic and Clinical Success in Field of Occupational Therapy: Predictors of Entry-Level Competence*. Unpublished doctoral dissertation. Philadelphia, PA: Temple University; 2003.
9. Zaccaro S, Rittman A, Marks M. Team leadership. *Leadersh Q*. 2001;12:451-483.
10. House R, Mitchell R. Path-goal theory of leadership. *J Contemp Bus*. 1974;3:81-97.
11. Masin, H. Education in the affective domain: a method/model for teaching professional behaviors in the classroom and during advisory session. *J Phys Ther Educ*. 2002;16:37-47.
12. Mostrom E. Professionalism in physical therapy: a reflection on ways of being in physical therapy education. *J Phys Ther Educ*. 2004;18:2-4.
13. McDonald C, Cox P, Bartlett D, Houghton P. Consensus on methods to foster physical therapy professional behaviors. *J Phys Ther Educ*. 2002;16:27-31.
14. Miller L, Bossers A, Polatajko HJ, Hartley M. Development of the competency based fieldwork evaluation (CBFE). *Occup Ther Int*. 2001;8(4):244-263.
15. Alsop A. Competence unfurled: developing portfolio practice. *Occup Ther Int*. 2001;8:126-132.
16. Gouveia W. The contemplative manager. *Am J Health Syst Pharm*. 2007;64:1299-1300.
17. McIvor O. The business of kindness—part 3: building leadership character traits. *AMT Events*. June 1, 2007:80-81.
18. Thomson L, Lieberman D, Murphy R, Wendt E, Poole J, Hertfelder S. *Developing, Maintaining, and Updating Competency in Occupational Therapy: A Guide to Self-Appraisal*. Bethesda, MD: American Occupational Therapy Association Press; 1995.
19. Christie B, Joyce P, Moeller P. Fieldwork experience, part I: impact on practice preference. *Am J Occup Ther*. 1985;39:671-674.
20. Haider E. Nurse leaders as teachers. *Nurs Manag*. 2007;14(4):30-33.
21. Hackman M, Johnson C. *Leadership: A Communication Perspective*. Prospect Heights, IL: Waveland Press; 2000.
22. Moody R, Horton-Deutsch S, Pesut D. Appreciative inquiry for leading in complex systems: supporting the transformation of academic nursing culture. *J Nurs Educ*. 2007;46(7):319-324.

23. Goleman D. What makes a leader? *Harv Bus Rev.* 2004;82(1):82-91.
24. Freshwater D, Stickley T. The heart of the art: Emotional intelligence in nurse education. *Nurs Inq.* 2004;11:91-98.
25. Goodfellow E. The potential of improved leadership sustainability within the new leadership paradigm. *Can J Respir Ther.* 2007;43(3):29-30.
26. May A, Norbury J. Follow the leader. *Emerg Nurs.* 2007;15(4):16-21.
27. Kerfoot K. The art of telling the truth: handling failures with disclosure and apology. *Dermatol Nurs.* 2007;19:298-300.

6

TEAMS AND OCCUPATIONAL THERAPY PRACTITIONER LEADERSHIP

Lesly S. Wilson, PhD, OTR/L

Learning Objectives

1. Identify a definition and purpose of a team versus a group.
2. Identify the types of teams and team approaches.
3. Understand stages of team development.
4. Describe the characteristics of effective teams.
5. Identify potential opportunities for occupational therapy practitioners in team leadership.
6. Apply team leadership to occupational therapy perspectives.

A leader leads by example, whether she intends to or not.
—Unknown Author

Defining Team Versus Group

Teams and Groups

A team is a group of interdependent individuals with complementary skills and a commitment to shared meaningful purpose, with specific goals.[1] The interdependence among individuals within teams is not present within a group. In a group, individuals interact with one another to maintain stable patterns of relationships and have common shared goals.[2] Group members are focused on individual outcomes and are often responsive to management from an individual perspective. The major difference between the 2 similar terms is that teams provide collective work products, individual and mutual accountability, and a common commitment to purpose with greater flexibility from management to do their job.

Today's health care organizations provide a variety of functions performed by numerous health care professionals, offering complex and specialized skills.[3] Occupational therapy practitioners are one group of health care professionals with specialized skills focused on enabling people to perform the day-to-day activities that are important to them despite impairments, activity limitations, participation restrictions, or risks of these problems.[4,5] Health care teams provide an opportunity to bring a variety of sophisticated skill and experience together for optimal patient outcome. Important implications for patient outcomes have been associated with the team process.[6]

This team process operates in a health care system that annually delivers 4 million babies; provides 762 million visits to physicians; enables 539 million days in the hospital; consumes about one-sixth of our income; and outpaces education, defense, welfare, pensions, and justice in spending.[7,8] The increase in cost of health care, hospital stays, government payments to the system, and total medical expenses have driven organizations to promote higher levels of efficiency and accountability. Teams are a common approach to address these concerns while providing avenues for holistic clinical decision making for health care consumers. However, one of the most critical challenges faced by organizations is team building.[1] There is limited focus toward team building or teamwork within clinical curriculum and training for health care professionals. The occupational therapy practitioners require academic preparation that focuses on aspects of marketing, leadership, strategic planning, and team building.[9]

The development of effective teams is critical from clinical and administrative perspectives. Nevertheless, it is important to understand that there are different types of teams employed within differing health care environments (Figure 6-1).

Types of Teams and Team Approaches

We are bound together by the task which lies before us.
—Martin Luther King

Team Types

Generally, teams are often categorized by 5 major dimensions[2]:

1. *Purpose or mission*: This dimension refers to the reason behind the formation of a team for a specific organizational purpose or mission. The formation of teams can be for a specific work project or a more ongoing improvement project. Work or improvement teams are under this dimension. Work teams are typically concerned with producing a product or a service, and they use the organization's resources to create results that are effective. Improvement teams are focused on the overall effectiveness of the organization's mission and purpose, and they look to create more effective processes within an organization.

2. *Time*: This dimension refers to the longevity of the team, which is typically based on the needs of the organization and includes temporary and permanent teams. Temporary teams are formed to accomplish specific tasks and are short-term. Permanent teams are formed to meet the ongoing needs of an organization and are long-term.

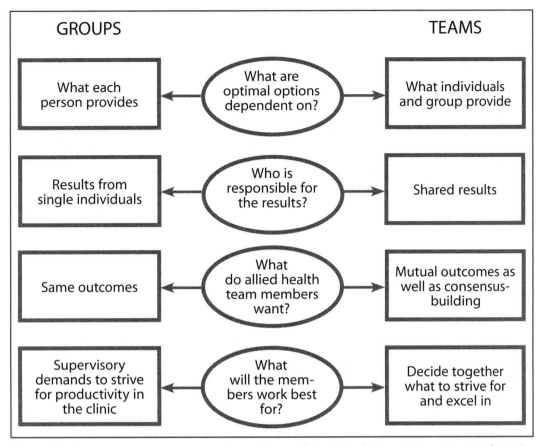

Figure 6-1. Group versus teams: a comparison. (Adapted from Greenberg J, Baron RA. Group dynamics and work teams. In: *Behavior in Organizations*. New Jersey: Pearson Prentice Hall; 2008:308.)

3. *Degree of autonomy*: This dimension refers to how a team is allowed to operate and focuses on the level of accountability and decision making of employees. Work groups and self-managed work teams are in this dimension. Work groups follow the leader, offering limited input to the decision-making process. Self-managed work teams are composed of a small number of employees to perform the duties of a supervisor.

4. *Authority structure*: This dimension refers to how a team is connected to the orga-nization's authority structure and includes intact and cross-functional teams. Intact teams work together continuously with expertise and skill in the same or similar areas. Cross-functional teams effectively bring together diverse expertise and skill from throughout an organization to work together on a common goal.

5. *Physical presence*: This dimension refers to how a team physically works together and includes physical and virtual teams. Physical teams involve people who physically meet to work together. Virtual teams operate across space, time, and organizational boundaries, fostering communication through technology.

General team structure is associated with the above dimensions. It is important to con-sider these dimensions as related to health care team development, structure, and opera-tion for a better understanding of team functionality within health care organizations. The understanding of such structural components can provide occupational therapy practitio-ners with a greater level of understanding concerning individual professional roles and responsibilities necessary to successfully operate as an effective team member (Figure 6-2).

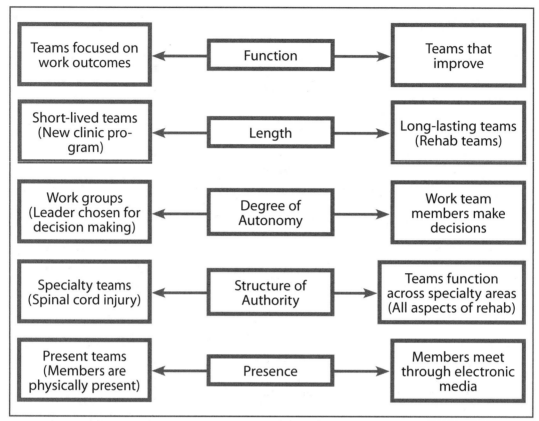

Figure 6-2. Types of teams. Adapted from Mohrman SA. Integrating roles and structure in the lateral organization. In: Galbraith JR, Lawler EE III, eds. *Organizing for the Future.* San Francisco: Jossey-Bass; 1993:109-141.

Team Approaches

Multidisciplinary, interdisciplinary, and transdisciplinary are the 3 team approaches. Each team approach should be matched with the appropriate health care environment, as each team approach may not work best in every health care environment.[10,11] Medical models typically have based teaming on multidisciplinary or interdisciplinary interaction.[12] However, these same models have been found problematic in community- and home-based service delivery settings.[13] Components such as authority structure, physical presence, patient diagnosis, and patient/family resources should be closely considered when determining a match of team type with health care environment, as it is these components that shape the levels of necessary interaction. Occupational therapy practitioners often operate within these team approaches during assessment, intervention, and discharge service delivery. They have working knowledge of these team approaches.

All 3 team approaches involve the contributions of team member expertise. However, the interactions among members differ greatly.

- Multidisciplinary teams are where professionals each work within their particular scope of practice and interact formally.[14] These team members perform evaluations independently, present evaluation findings to other team members, and offer no or limited formal interaction among some team members. Occupational therapy practitioners typically encounter these teams in private or hospital outpatient settings.

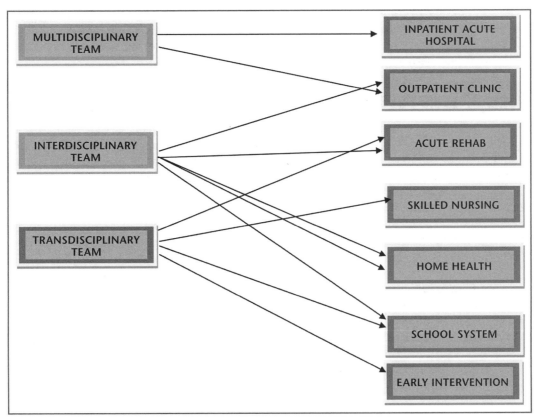

Figure 6-3. Team approaches and settings. Suggested approach and treatment setting matches by Lesly S. Wilson.

- Interdisciplinary teams are characterized by a greater overlapping of professional roles, formal and informal communication, and shared problem solving for the good of the patient.[14] These team members complete evaluations independently, share and discuss evaluation findings with other team members, and have formal interaction with other team members regarding consumer health care needs. Occupational therapy practitioners are possibly most familiar and comfortable within these team environments as they are representative of acute rehabilitation inpatient settings and skilled nursing facilities that employ large numbers of occupational therapy practitioners.

- Transdisciplinary teams provide greater blending (or blurring) of roles.[14] It is based on collaboration, consensus building, and role release among professionals from differing theoretical and specialty backgrounds. Transdisciplinary teams conduct evaluations together as a team, incorporate appropriate methods from all disciplines in evaluations, and share and discuss evaluation findings with all team members. Role release and role expansion are challenges that occupational therapy practitioners typically encounter within transdisciplinary teaming. Occupational therapy practitioners frequently are experiencing this teaming approach more in early intervention and school settings. Figure 6-3 pairs team approaches with typical settings for a clearer understanding of common relationships and occupational therapy practitioner involvement.

It is important to note that within some settings, multiple team approaches may be employed to best serve the individual needs of a client. These team approaches should be carefully studied with thoughtful determination concerning which approach works best for which treatment setting or individual patient case.

Model of Team Development

The formation of effective and high-performing teams is a process that evolves over a period of time. Bruce Tuckman's stage model of group development, published in 1965, remains one of the most commonly cited models of group development today.[15-17] This model categorizes group development into 5 distinct stages. Each stage is a prerequisite for moving into the next stage, with recommendations that no stage is skipped during the process. Skipping stages may hinder the overall development and performance of a team. Forming, storming, norming, performing, and adjourning are the 5 stages of group development, illustrated in Figure 6-4.

1. *Forming* is the initial stage Tuckman suggests in group development. This initial stage involves team members coming together, introducing themselves to one another, making character observations, and getting to know one another. In health care teams, this stage may involve clinical and administrative disciplines discussing scopes of practice, experiences, and interest. This stage often comes with team member uncertainty, lack of trust, anxiety, and avoidance of conflict. The stage involves directing on the part of the team leader. The team leader should provide clear directives concerning team purpose, objectives, and goals while directing the roles and responsibilities of team members. This is a time for occupational therapy practitioners to learn more about other disciplines' scope of practice and experience and to determine collaborative treatment opportunities. Following the forming stage is a natural flow into the storming stage of team development.

2. *Storming* is a stage associated with team conflict, confusion of roles or responsibilities, and the organization of the team. Continued discussion of roles and responsibilities occurs in this stage. In health care teams, this stage may involve disagreements with team member roles and responsibilities as related to specific patient cases. This stage comes with resistance and hostility toward other team members and the team leader. The team leader should make attempts to discuss areas of conflict and confusion while fostering negation and consensus on issues of concern. This is a time for occupational therapy practitioners to educate other disciplines on the broad scope of occupational therapy practice, stand firm for suggestive treatment planning or implemented approaches, and display their psychological skill within the team. It is often an unsteady and challenging stage of team development. However, it is followed by the norming stage.

3. *Norming* is the stage where team members begin to develop a better understanding of roles and responsibilities along with tasks. Norms and ground rules of engagement are established and agreed upon. In health care teams, this stage may involve team members clearing their understanding of each other's clinical and administrative training and experiences. It is also a time where appreciation of health care team member roles and responsibilities becomes clear. The team leader becomes more of a facilitator, allowing team members to develop cohesiveness and a stronger group structure. This is a time when occupational therapy practitioners have developed a greater understanding of team member professional disciplines, appreciation of roles and responsibilities, and clinical experiences. It is often the stage of group development where the team members and leader begin to settle down prior to transitioning into the performing stage.

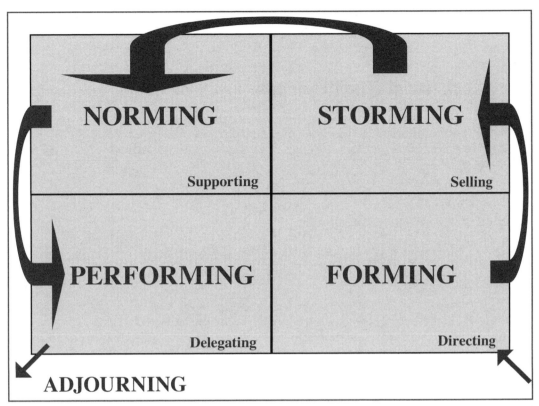

Figure 6-4. The 5 stages of group development. (Copyright 1965 by the American Psychological Association. Reprinted with permission. This information appeared in an article in *Psychological Bulletin*, Volume 63, Number 6, Pages 384-399.)

4. *Performing* is the stage where team members begin functioning well together and working toward their team-intended purpose. In health care teams, this stage may involve team members functioning appropriately within multidisciplinary, interdisciplinary, and transdisciplinary approaches. This stage is when the team works smoothly and efficiently with their members and leaders. There is great loyalty, respect, and appreciation of team members during this phase. This is a time when occupational therapy practitioners can display their clinical and leadership skills to other team members, as well as develop a greater appreciation of the other team members. It is the final stage of team development before moving into adjourning.

5. *Adjourning* was a fifth stage added by Tuckman 10 years after the unveiling of the initial 4 stages of team development. This stage occurs when teams end or conclude their purpose or when team members disengage themselves. In health care teams, this stage may not be present for all teams. This is a time when occupational therapy practitioners can display skill in discharge planning, control of resources, and initiative to ensure that the most optimal continuum of care is recommended for a patient. It is important to refer to the team types and dimensions of the team to determine if this stage will be inclusive of a health care team process. For example, temporary team types may more commonly evolve to this stage over permanent team types.

It is important to realize that not all teams transition from one stage to the next smoothly, and some teams spend longer timeframes in one stage over others. There are additional processes related to the occupational therapy practitioner that should be considered during each phase of the team-building processes. Some teams also slip back into the storming stage after having transitioned into the norming stage. Other teams never evolve to the performing stage. They are disbanded or discouraged prior to transition into the performing stage.

Characteristics of Effective Teams

Effective teams have a clear understanding of purpose and objectives. They operate within their organizational framework of mission, purpose, and objectives.

Effective teams have 7 characteristics that can best be described by the acronym PERFORM[19]:

1. Purpose and values

2. Empowerment

3. Relationships and communication

4. Flexibility

5. Optimal performance

6. Recognition and appreciation

7. Morale

Mixtures of these characteristics frequently result in high-performing teams within organizations. Such effective teams exhibit a clearly defined and agreed-upon purpose with common values. The team goals are plainly communicated and understood. The team is empowered to make decisions and take necessary actions to enforce the agreed decisions. It presents cultural and diversity concerns respectfully while encouraging differing perspectives and opinions. Effective teams turn mistakes into opportunities while using the expertise of each team member. They are open to exploring new approaches and strategies for handling challenges. These teams are continuously seeking to improve their efforts while producing significant results. The team members of effective teams acknowledge individual member and team accomplishments. They are confident, with a strong sense of pride and satisfaction in the produced work.

Effective teams utilize quality improvement in decision-making processes to assist with developing their team procedures, services, or products to their satisfaction level. The Shewhart Cycle is often employed by effective teams to guide improvement processes.[20] This cycle is commonly referred to as the Plan-Do-Check-Act Cycle (PDCA) or the Deming Cycle. It has been found useful to assist team problem-solving processes (Figure 6-5).

Effective teams employ a systematic problem-solving process, as outlined in the 4-step PDCA Cycle. This checklist-type of approach fosters thorough review and thought toward problems. It allows adequate team thought and input toward problem solving. The Plan phase identifies the team problem or concern while developing ideas to address each problem. The Do phase implements the plan decided upon during the Plan phase. The Check phase evaluates the outcomes from the implemented plan in the Do phase. The Act phase allows for implementation of plan on a more global perspective within an organization. The PDCA Cycle is a process that can be applied to various problems for systematic review and continuous quality improvement.

Occupational therapy practitioner team members and leaders should be aware of such models of effective team development and operation. They should note these common characteristics of effective teams and employ systematic problem solving and continuous quality improvement to ensure effective health care team decision making. Awareness of these characteristics can help these team members and leaders better identify whether they are operating effectively and understand how to operate more effectively.

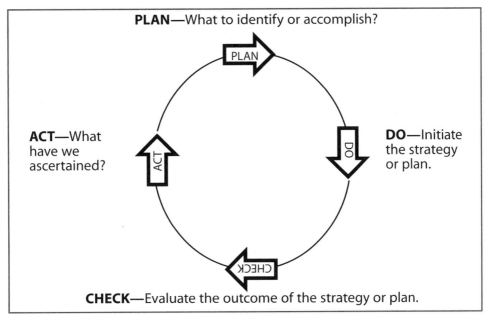

Figure 6-5. Plan-Do-Act-Check Cycle. Created by Jim Winings. Reproduced with permission from http://www.sixsigmaspc.com/dictionary/PDCA-plan-do-check-act.html.

Team Leadership and Occupational Therapy Practitioners

If your actions inspire others to dream more, learn more,
do more, and become more, you are a leader.
—John Quincy Adams

Teams require leadership to be successful. Leadership has been coined as an art and has been questioned as being a born characteristic over a learned characteristic. It has been defined as the ability to convince people to follow a path they have never taken before to a place they have never been, and upon finding it to be successful, convincing them to do it over and over again.[21] Leadership involves making things that appear to be impossible or not thought to be possible possible. According to Colin Powell, "Leadership is the art of accomplishing more than the science of management says is possible."[22] The health care industry has emerged into a new creature that includes advanced technology, logistics, strategic plans, workforce diversity, workplace diversity, and much more. This evolution of change requires effective team work and leadership. Organizations are challenged to identify employees with leadership skills. They are being forced to hire, promote, and produce employees with leadership potential while being encumbered with rules, regulations, and traditions.

Health care teams require leaders with a style that allows for flexibility as environments, patient needs, and team compositions all differ. Situational leadership is a common style of team leaders. Situational leadership provides direction or autocratic behavior and support or democratic behavior.[19] This theory provides the best leadership style for a given situation and has been considered a contingency theory. Situational leaders should be able to diagnose the situations they face, identify the appropriate behavioral style, and then implement that response.[23] Occupational therapy practitioner leaders who are able to lead teams during given situations will be more successful in dynamic health care environments.

As situational leaders, occupational therapy practitioners should possess transformational leadership. Transformational leadership "links leaders and followers in a relationship characterized not only by power, but also by mutual needs, aspirations, and values known as moral leadership."[24] This leadership raises consciousness by articulating and modeling clear values and vision.[25] Occupational therapy practitioners who are able to exhibit transformational leadership will act as change agents by changing the tide or course of events within health care teams and organizations.

Opportunities for occupational therapy practitioners have increased, and these trained clinicians must be ready to meet the challenge as such opportunities evolve.[26] Operating as situational leaders allows occupational therapy practitioners to exhibit such dynamic leadership behaviors as guiding, clarifying, collaborating, and fulfilling during the team process. Occupational therapy practitioners have skills in task analysis and can utilize this skill in team situations to further their leadership roles.

Applying the Occupational Therapy Practice Framework in Teams

The *Occupational Therapy Practice Framework: Domain and Process*[27,28] can be applied to clinical team processes. This framework clearly outlines a process for occupational therapy practice, which can be applied to foster leadership in team situations. The overarching domain of occupational therapy practice is "supporting health and participation in life through engagement on occupation."[28] Focusing on this outcome throughout the process of practice will help to ensure that interventions are within the profession's domain.[29] The initial step in the practice framework process is evaluation. During the evaluation process, an occupational profile of the client's history, experiences, patterns of daily living, interests, values, and needs are established by the occupational therapy practitioner.[29] This same concept can be applied in the team development forming stage. An occupational profile of a team member's clinical or administrative background, strengths, interest, values, and needs can be established by the occupational therapy practitioner. Such information will help the practitioner better understand the roles, responsibilities, and interest of other team members. As a team leader, such information will help occupational therapy practitioners to better guide the team process through tasks by having a clearer understanding of other professional's clinical background, experience, and interest.

The next step outlined in the practice framework process is intervention. This step includes intervention planning, intervention implementation, and intervention review.[29] This same concept can be applied in the team development storming and norming stages. During these team development stages, occupational therapy practitioners should be active in the planning related to the client's overall functional outcomes, be suggestive with interventions for implementation, and actively participate in the evaluation of the intervention plan developed by the team. The storming and norming stage processes allow for the occupational therapy practitioners to share the global perspectives that impact consumers' activities of daily living and interact with team members to develop the most optimal plan of care. As a team leader, active involvement in planning, implementation, and intervention helps foster the clarifying and collaboration behavior necessary to lead the team through tasks.

The final step outlined in the practice framework is outcome. This step focuses on consistently helping clients to achieve the fullest possible participation in their families, schools, work settings, and communities.[29] This same concept can be applied to the team development performing stage. During this stage, occupational therapy practitioners should ensure that individual discipline goals or outcomes are achieved as well as team outcomes. The success of the team process should be most apparent during the performing stage as it is when true teamwork efforts should prevail. The adjourning stage of team development should also be associated with the outcome phase of the practice framework. This stage is when the team disbands itself or ends a current project. This same concept can be applied in the outcome phase. As each client is served and reaches his or her most optimal potential, the team composition may decrease or the entire team may end its work with the client.

The occupational therapy practice framework provides an applicable guide for team involvement and leadership that should be embraced by practitioners. These concepts of practice are transferable and should be utilized to help occupational therapy practitioners become leaders within team environments.

Summary

Teams will continue to function within health care as they provide an avenue for providing consumers of health services the most optimal care. It is important that occupational therapy practitioners have a clear understanding of the differences between a team and a group, as well as understand the stages of team development. In order for occupational therapy practitioners to propel into leadership within health care organizations, a clear operational understanding of team development and experience with teamwork will be necessary.

Case Example

Billy, a 56-year-old male with a cerebral vascular accident (CVA), has been admitted to an acute rehab facility. The occupational therapist has performed a complete assessment with findings that indicate that Billy's deficits include flaccidity in left arm with left-sided neglect, poor strength in left leg for ambulation, poor dynamic balance for tasks at standing, and mild memory losses. He is a chef, has a wife and 3 children, and would like to return home and be able to continue to participate as a coach with his son's soccer team. The newly hired occupational therapy practitioner will serve as a rehab team member for Billy's case.

1. Following the AOTA 2008 *Occupational Therapy Practice Framework: Domain and Process* and Tuckman's *Five Stages of Team Development*, what should some initial steps be for the occupational therapy practitioner and why?

2. During a future rehab team meeting, the administrator suggests that the team consider discharging Billy from the facility prior to when the team-agreed plan of care is completed. The occupational, physical, and speech therapist are outraged and begin pleading the case for Billy to stay the full length of time necessary. What stage of team development does this most closely represent and why?

3. Billy shows improvement in at least one goal from occupational, physical, and speech therapy at the rehab team meeting. What stage of team development does this most closely represent and why?

4. Billy has achieved all occupational therapy and physical therapy goals with some speech goals improved but not fully achieved by the rehab team meeting. The administrator suggests discharging Billy with home health services to continue working on speech deficit areas. What stage of team development does this most closely represent and why?

Reflection Activity

1. What is the difference between a team and a group?
2. Identify and discuss the 5 dimensions of team types.
3. Identify and discuss differences of team approaches.
4. What are the 5 stages of team development?
5. What is the purpose of a team charter?
6. Why is the PDCA Cycle important in the team process?
7. What is situational leadership?
8. How can the occupational therapy practice framework process be utilized within the team development process?

References

1. Payne V. *The Team-Building Workshop: A Trainer's Guide*. New York, NY: Amacom; 2001.
2. Greenberg J, Baron RA. *Behavior in Organizations*. 9th ed. Upper Saddle River, NJ: Pearson Prentice Hall; 2008.
3. McConnell CR. The manager and continuing education. *The Health Care Manager*. 2002. 21(2), 72-84.
4. Christiansen C, Baum C. *Occupational Therapy: Enabling Function and Wellbeing*. Thorofare, NJ: SLACK Incorporated; 1997.
5. Neistadt ME, Crepeau EB, eds. *Willard & Spackman's Occupational Theapy*. 9th ed. Philadelphia, PA: Lippincott Williams & Wilkins; 1998.
6. Alexander JA, Lichtenstein R, Jinnett K, Wells R, Zazzali J, Liu D. Cross functional team processes and patient functional improvement. *Health Serv Res*. 2005;40(5):1335-1355.
7. Griffin JR. *The Well-Managed Healthcare Organization*. 4th ed. Chicago, IL: Health Administration Press; 1999.
8. Elliot N, Quinless F. The future in healthcare delivery. *Nurs Health Care Perspect*. 2000;21(2):84-92.
9. McCormack GL. Occupational therapy skills and management skills. In: McCormack GL, Jaffe EG, Goodman-Lavey M, eds. *OT Manager*. 4th ed. Bethesda, MD: American Occupational Therapy Association Press; 2003:23-32.
10. Paul S, Peterson CQ. Interprofessional collaboration: issues for practice and research. *Occup Ther Health Care*. 2001;15(3/4):1-12.
11. Weiland D, Kramer BJ, Waite MS, Rubenstein LZ. The interdisciplinary team in geriatric care. *Am Behav Sci*. 1996;39(6):655-664.
12. Bergen D, Wright M. Medical assessment perspectives. In: Bergen D, ed. *Assessment Methods for Infants and Toddlers: Transdisciplinary Team Approaches*. New York, NY: Teachers College Press; 1994:40-56.
13. Stephans MB, Thompson CL, Buchanan ML. The role of the nurse on a transdisciplinary early intervention assessment team. *Public Health Nurs*. 2002;19(4):238-245.
14. Sheehan D, Robertson L, Ormond T. Comparison of language used and patterns of communication in interprofessional and multidisciplinary teams. *J Interprof Care*. 2007;21(1):17-30.
15. Cissna K. Phases in group development. *Small Croup Behavior*. 1984:15;3-32.
16. Smith MK, Bruce W, Tuckman. Forming, storming, norming and performing in groups. 2005. In the Encyclopedia of informed education. Available at: http://www.infed.org/thinkers/tuckman.htm.
17. Worchel S. You can go home again: returning group research to the group context with an eye on development issues. *Small Croup Research*. 1994:25;205-224.
18. Blanchard, K, Carew, D, & Parisi. *High Five! The Magic of Working Together*. New York, NY: HarperCollins Publishers; 2001.
19. Blanchard K, Carew D, Parisi-Carew E. *The One-Minute Manager Builds High Performing Teams*. New York, NY: HarperCollins Publishers; 2000.
20. Griffith JR, White KR. *The Well-Managed Healthcare Organization*. 6th ed. Chicago, IL: Health Administration Press; 2007.
21. Mariotti J. On management: the role of a leader. 1999. Available at: http://www.industryweek.com/articles/on_management_the_role_of_a_leader-_1753.aspx. Accessed June 30, 2009.
22. McGowan P. Management vs. leadership (development of administrator's leadership skills in school reform). 2001. Available at: http://www.findarticles.com/of_o/mOJSD/10_58/79628950/print.jhtml. Accessed March 25, 2002.
23. Greenberg J. *Managing Behavior in Organizations*. 4th ed. Upper Saddle River, NJ: Pearson Prentice Hall; 2005.
24. Grady AP. From management to leadership. In: McCormack GL, Jaffe EG, Goodman-Lavey M, eds. *OT Manager*. 4th ed. Bethesda, MD: American Occupational Therapy Association Press; 2003:331-347.

25. Astin A, Astin H. *Leadership Reconsidered: Engaging Higher Education in Social Change.* Battle Creek, MI: W.K. Kellogg Foundation; 2000.
26. Bravemen BH. Staff development systems: effective strategies for professional growth. *Administration & Management Special Interest Section Quarterly.* 2001;17(1):1-3.
27. American Occupational Therapy Association. Occupational therapy practice framework: domain and process. *Am J Occup Ther.* 2002;56:609-639.
28. American Occupational Therapy Association. Occupational therapy practice framework: domain and process. 2nd ed. *Am J Occup Ther.* 2008;62:625-683.
29. LaVesser P, Davidson DA. The occupational therapy practice framework: domain and process applied to a client with developmental disabilities. *Dev Disabil Spec Interest Sect Q.* 2004;27:1-3.

Index

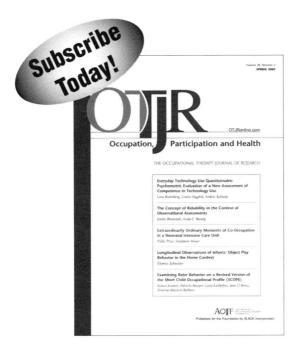

OTJR: Occupation, Participation and Health
ISSN# 1539-4492

OTJR: Occupation, Participation and Health offers original research articles that advance the knowledge of occupational therapy practice and an understanding of the role occupation plays in fostering personal well-being, enabling full participation in the community, and enhancing the health of individuals and society.

Inside you'll find:

- Research briefs
- Original articles
- Commentaries
- Letters to the editor

Contact SLACK Incorporated for pricing details.

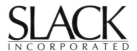

SLACK Incorporated • Health Care Books and Journals
6900 Grove Road • Thorofare, NJ 08086

1-800-257-8290 or 1-856-848-1000

Fax: 1-856-848-6091 • E-mail: customerservice@slackinc.com • Visit: www.OTJRonline.com

DATE DUE

Demco, Inc. 38-293